The Ultimate Vegetarian Dish Cookbook

Easy And Healthy Vegetarian Recipes For Beginners

Riley Bloom

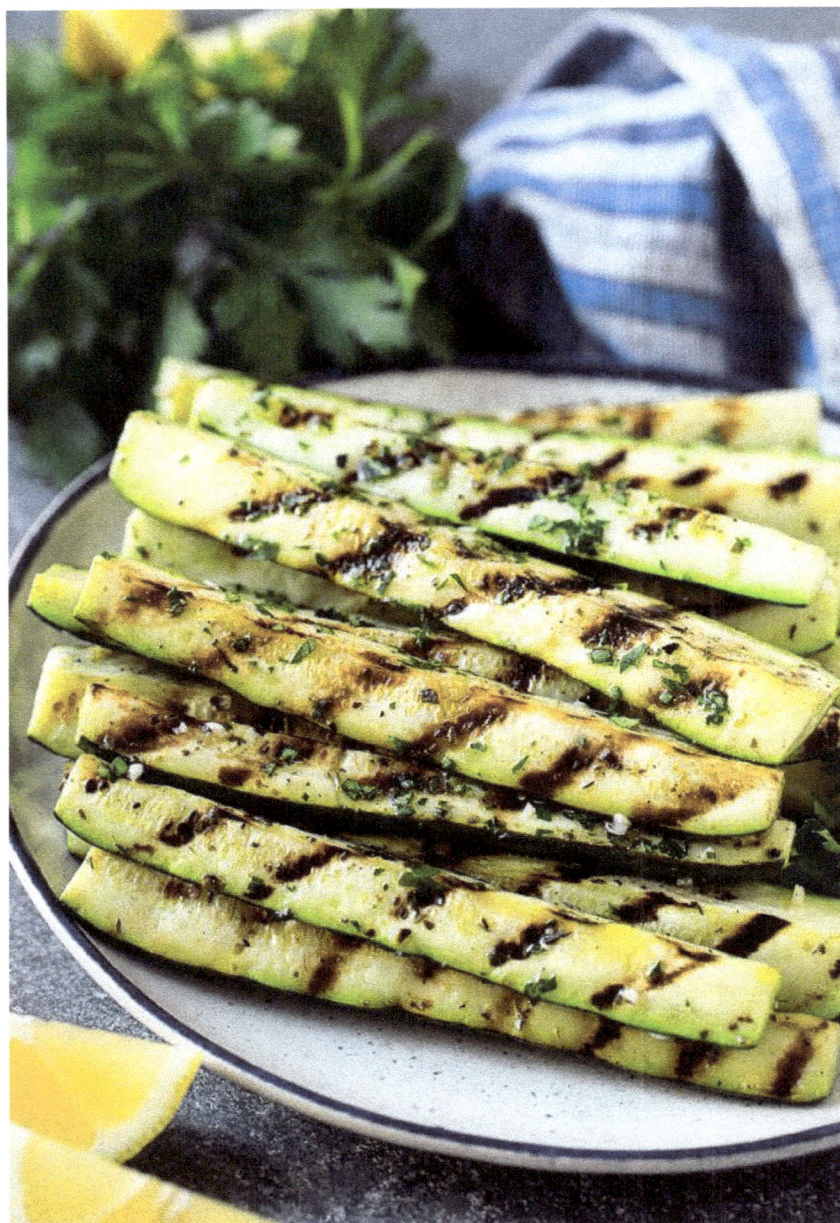

Table of contents

Kidney Beans & Button Mushrooms with Pesto Sauce 7

Slow Cooked Quinoa and Tomatoes 9

Black Rice with Enoki Mushroom in Chimichurri..................... 11

Quinoa and Enoki Mushrooms 13

Brown Rice with Vegan Chorizo and Ancho Chili.....................15

Split Pea Celery and Leek Soup.....................17

Slow Cooked Chick Peas and Vegetarian Sausage 19

Red Potato and Baby Spinach Soup 22

Grilled Zucchinis and Crimini Mushrooms...................... 24

Grilled Asparagus Carrots and Squash Marinade.....................27

Grilled Sweet Corns and Portobello...................... 30

Grilled Bell Pepper and Broccolini 33

Grilled Corn and Crimini Mushrooms 34

Grilled Zucchini and Pineapple......................37

Grilled Asparagus and Mushrooms 39

Grilled Japanese Eggplant Bell Peppers and Broccolini 40

Grilled Japanese Bell Pepper and Cauliflower Recipe with Balsamic Glaze
.... 43

Grilled Eggplant and Yellow Bell Peppers...................... 44

Grilled Collard Greens and Portobello Mushrooms 47

Red Cabbage and Onion in Ranch Dressing 49

Grilled Broccolini Asparagus and Eggplants.....................51

Grilled Rutabaga and Mustard Greens 54

Grilled Turnips with Broccoli 57

Grilled Turnip and Beetroots 60

Grilled Water Chestnuts and Mangoes 62

Grilled Artichoke Hearts and Water Chestnuts 65

Grilled Assorted Bell Peppers with Broccolini Florets Recipe ... 66

Grilled Portobello and Rutabaga 67

Grilled Brussel Sprouts Cauliflower and Rutabaga 70

Grilled Water Chestnuts Swiss Chard and Asparagus Recipe 71

Grilled Asparagus Pineapple and Green Beans 72

Asparagus Dressing 74

Grilled Broccoli & Swiss Chard 76

Grilled Water Chestnuts and Green Beans 77

Grilled Turnip Greens and Okra 78

Grilled Beetroots and Purple Cabbage 81

Grilled Turnip and Endives 84

Grilled Green Beans and Pineapple 85

Grilled Turnip and Zucchini 87

Grilled Portobello Mushrooms and Broccolini Florets 89

Grilled Beetroots and Artichoke Hearts 91

Grilled Baby Carrots and Zucchini 94

Grilled Water Chestnuts Baby Carrots and Artichoke Hearts 96

Grilled Rutabaga Zucchini and Onions 97

Grilled Rutabaga Broccolini Florets and Bell Peppers 100

5

Grilled Baby Carrots and Winter Squash 101

Grilled Beetroots and Artichoke Hearts in Viniagrette 104

Grilled Beetroots Artichoke Hearts and Asparagus...................................105

Grilled Summer Squash with Balsamic Glaze... 106

Kidney Beans & Button Mushrooms with Pesto Sauce

Ingredients

- 2 red onions
- 7 garlic cloves
- 1 ancho chili, minced
- 1 tbsp. lime juice
- 4 cups vegetable broth
- 1 can water (I use the can of diced tomatoes to grab all the leftover flavor)
- 8 oz. dried kidney beans
- 1 15 oz can button mushrooms
- 3 tablespoons pesto sauce
- 1 teaspoons dried basil, coarsely chopped
- 1 tsp. dried Italian seasoning
- 1/2 cup uncooked rice
- 1/4 teaspoon sea salt

Directions:

Put all of the ingredients into slow cooker. Cook on low for 8 hours or high for 4 hours. Serve with toppings such as shredded vegan cheese, avocado, green onion and cilantro

Slow Cooked Quinoa and Tomatoes

Ingredients

- 1 red onion, chopped 1 white onion, chopped

- 8 garlic cloves, minced

- 1 tsp. shallot, minced

- 1 15 oz can diced tomatoes

- 4 cups vegetable broth

- 1 can water (I use the can of diced tomatoes to grab all the leftover flavor)

- 2 15 oz cans sliced porcini mushrooms

- 2 tablespoons chili powder

- 2 teaspoons cumin
  1 tablespoon oregano

- 1/2 cup uncooked quinoa

- 1/4 teaspoon sea salt

Directions:

Put all of the ingredients into slow cooker. Cook on low for 8 hours or high for 4 hours. Serve with toppings such as shredded vegan cheese, avocado, green onion and cilantro

Black Rice with Enoki Mushroom in Chimichurri

Ingredients

- 2 red onions

- 7 garlic cloves

- 1 ancho chili, minced

- 1 tbsp. lime juice

- 1 15 oz can diced tomatoes

- 4 cups vegetable broth
  1 can water (I use the can of diced tomatoes to grab all the leftover flavor)

- 1 8 oz can enoki mushrooms

- 2 tablespoons garlic, minced

- 2 teaspoons chili powder

- 1 tablespoon chimichurri

- 1/2 cup uncooked black rice

- 1/4 teaspoon sea salt

Directions:

Put all of the ingredients into slow cooker. Cook on low for 8 hours or high for 4 hours. Serve with toppings such as shredded vegan cheese, avocado, green onion and cilantro

Quinoa and Enoki Mushrooms

Ingredients

- 2 red onion, chopped

- 7 garlic cloves, minced

- 8 jalapeno peppers, minced

- 1 tbsp. lemon juice

- 4 cups vegetable broth

- 1 can water (I use the can of diced tomatoes to grab all the leftover flavor)

- 1 15 oz can enoki mushrooms

- 1 15 oz can button mushrooms

- 2 tablespoons chili powder

- 2 teaspoons cumin

- 1 tablespoon oregano

- 1/2 cup uncooked quinoa

- 1/4 teaspoon sea salt

Directions:

Put all of the ingredients into slow cooker. Cook on low for 8 hours or high for 4 hours. Serve with toppings such as shredded vegan cheese, avocado, green onion and cilantro

Brown Rice with Vegan Chorizo and Ancho Chili

Ingredients

- 2 red onions

- 7 garlic cloves

- 1 ancho chili, minced

- 1 tbsp. lime juice

- 4 cups vegetable broth

- 1 can water (I use the can of diced tomatoes to grab all the leftover flavor)

- 1 cup crimini mushrooms

- 1/2 cup vegan Chorizo (Soyrizo), crumbled

- 2 tablespoons annatto seeds

- 2 teaspoons cumin

- 1 tsp. cayenne pepper

- 1/2 cup uncooked brown rice

- 1/4 teaspoon sea salt

Directions:

Put all of the ingredients into slow cooker. Cook on low for 8 hours or high for 4 hours. Serve with toppings such as shredded vegan cheese, avocado, green onion and cilantro

Split Pea Celery and Leek Soup

Ingredients

- 1 16- oz package

- 1 lb dried green split peas, rinsed

- 1 large leek light green and white portion only, chopped and thoroughly cleaned

- 3 celery ribs diced

- 2 large carrots diced

- 4 garlic clove minced

- 1/4 cup chopped fresh parsley

- 6 cups vegetable broth

- 1/2 t ground black pepper

- 1 tsp sea salt or to taste

- 1 bay leaf

Directions:

Pour all of the ingredients in a slow cooker and combine thoroughly. Cover a cook on low heat for 7 and a half hours or high 3 and a half hours. Take out the bay leaf.

Slow Cooked Chick Peas and Vegetarian Sausage

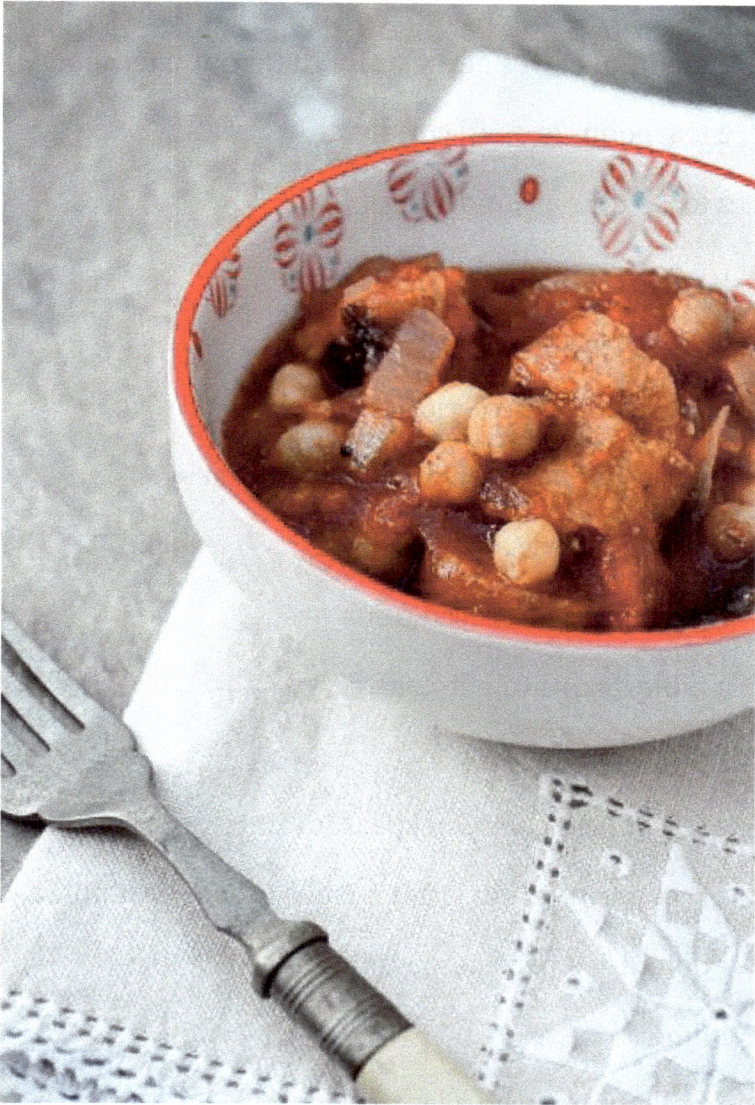

Ingredients

- 2 teaspoons extra virgin olive oil
- 1 medium red onion, diced (about 2 cups)
- 4 medium cloves garlic, minced (about 2 teaspoons)
- 2 teaspoons ground coriander
- 2 teaspoons ground cumin
- 1/2 teaspoon garam masala
- 1/2 teaspoon ground ginger
- 1/4 teaspoon turmeric
- 1/4 teaspoon crushed red pepper flakes
- 1 teaspoon sea salt
- 1 (15-ounce) can diced tomatoes
- 2 tablespoons tomato paste
- 1 cup vegetable stock
- 2 (15-ounce) cans chickpeas, drained and rinsed
- 1/2 cup vegetarian grain meat sausages, crumble
- 1 pound red potatoes, cut into 1/2-inch dice
- 1 lime
- Small bunch fresh cilantro

Equipment:

- 3-quart or larger slow cooker

Directions:

Heat the olive oil in a large pan over medium heat. Sauté the onion until softened and translucent. This takes about 5 minutes. Add in the garlic, coriander, cumin, garam masala, ground ginger, turmeric, red pepper flakes, and sea salt. Cook and stir for 1 minute. Add in the diced tomatoes, tomato paste, and vegetable broth. Combine and pour into the slow cooker. Add the chickpeas and potatoes. Cook on high heat for 4 1/2 hours or low for 9 hours, or until the potatoes become fork-tender. Serve in bowls and garnished with fresh cilantro and lime wedges

Red Potato and Baby Spinach Soup

Ingredients

- 5 cups low sodium vegetable stock

- 3 large red potatoes peeled and chopped

- 1 cup onion chopped

- 2 stalks celery chopped

- 4 cloves garlic crushed

- 1 cup heavy cream

- 1 tsp. dried tarragon

- 2 cups baby spinach

- 6-8 tbsp. sliced almonds

- sea salt and ground black pepper to taste

Directions:

Combine stock, sweet potatoes, onion, celery, and garlic to a 4-quart slow cooker. Cook on low heat for 8 hours or until potatoes become soft. Add almond milk, tarragon, salt and pepper. Blend this mixture for 1-2 minutes with an immersion blender until soup is smooth. Add baby spinach & cover. Let it rest for 20 minutes or until spinach becomes soft. Garnish with almonds and season with sea salt and pepper.

Grilled Zucchinis and Crimini Mushrooms

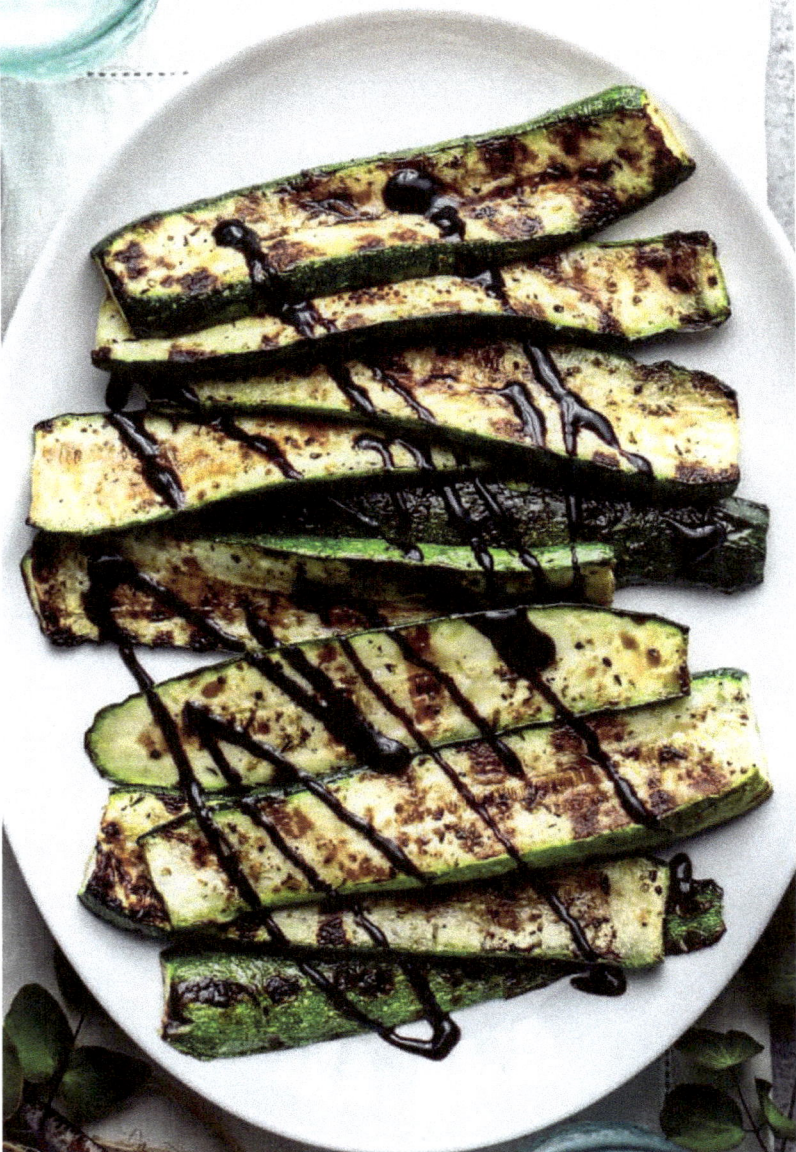

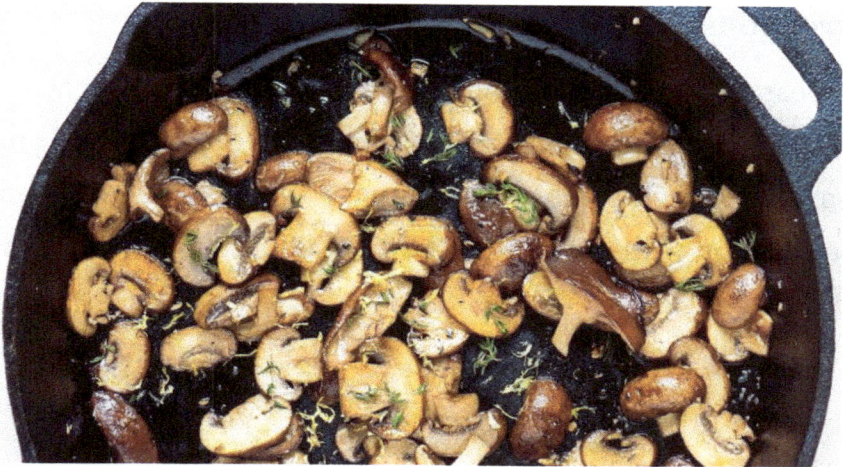

Ingredients

- 2 zucchinis, cut into 1/2-inch slices

- 2 red bell peppers, cut into chunks

- 1/2 pound fresh crimini mushrooms

- 1/2 pound cherry tomatoes

- 1 red onion, cut into 1/2-inch-thick slices

- 1/2 cup olive oil sea salt to taste

- Freshly ground black pepper to taste

Directions:

Preheat your grill for medium-high heat Oil the grate. Mix the zucchinis, green bell peppers, mushrooms, tomatoes, and onion in a bowl. Drizzle some olive oil over vegetables and toss them to coat. Season with sea salt and pepper. Grill the vegetables for 4 minutes per side.

Grilled Asparagus Carrots and Squash Marinade

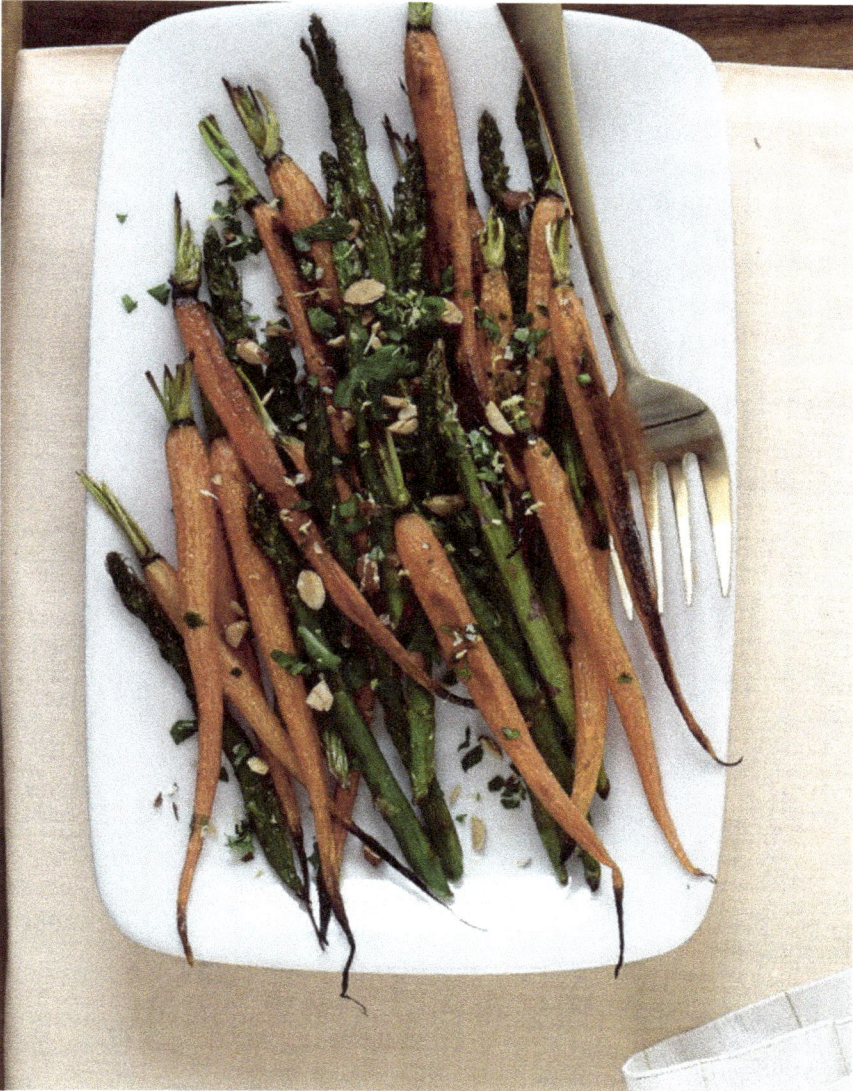

Ingredients

- 1/4 cup extra virgin olive oil
- 2 tablespoons honey
- 4 teaspoons balsamic vinegar
- 1 teaspoon dried oregano
- 1 teaspoon garlic powder
- 1/8 teaspoon rainbow peppercorns
- Sea salt

Vegetable Ingredients

- 1 pound fresh asparagus, trimmed
- 3 small carrots, cut in half lengthwise
- 1 large sweet green pepper, cut into 1-inch strips
- 1 medium yellow summer squash, cut into 1/2-inch slices
- 1 medium yellow onion, cut into wedges

Directions:

Combine the marinade ingredients. Combine the 3 tablespoons marinade and vegetables in a bag.

Marinate 1 1/2 hours at room temperature or overnight in the refrigerator. Grill the vegetables over medium heat for 8-12 minutes or until tender. Sprinkle the remaining marinade.

Grilled Sweet Corns and Portobello

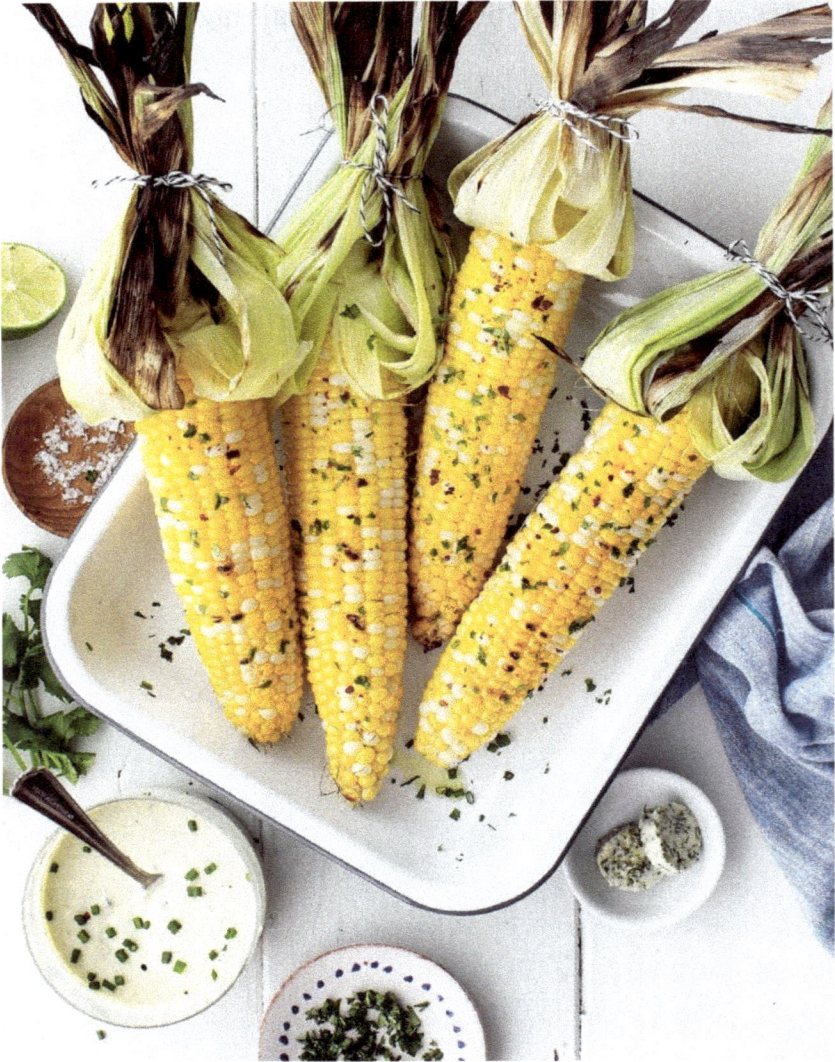

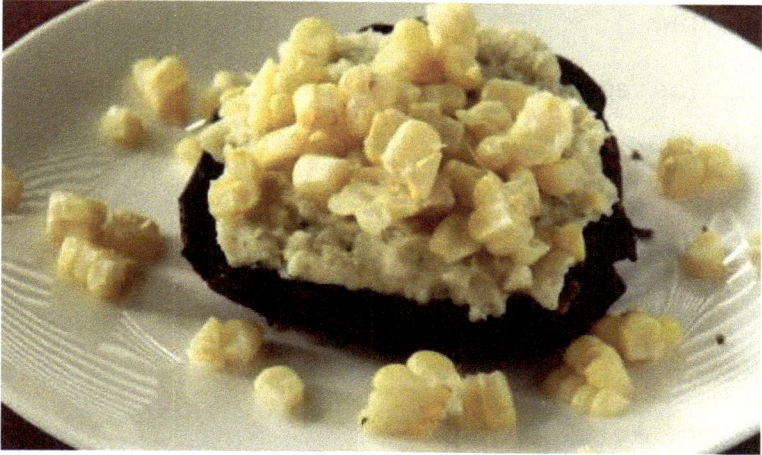

Ingredients

- 2 large Sweet Corns, cut lengthwise

- 5 pcs. Portobello, rinsed and drained

Marinade

- 6 tbsp. extra virgin olive oil

- Sea salt, to taste

- 3 tbsp.distilled white vinegar

- 1 tsp. Dijon mustard

Directions:

Marinate the vegetable with the dressing or marinade ingredients for 15 to 30 min. Grill for 4 minutes over medium heat or until the vegetable becomes tender.

Grilled Bell Pepper and Broccolini

Ingredients

- 2 green Bell Peppers, cut in half
- 10 Broccolini Florets

Marinade Ingredients:

- 6 tbsp. extra virgin olive oil
- Sea salt, to taste
- 3 tbsp. distilled white vinegar
- 1 tsp. sun-dried tomato pesto sauce

Directions:

Marinate the vegetable with the dressing or marinade ingredients for 15 to 30 min. Grill for 4 minutes over medium heat or until the vegetable becomes tender.

Grilled Corn and Crimini Mushrooms

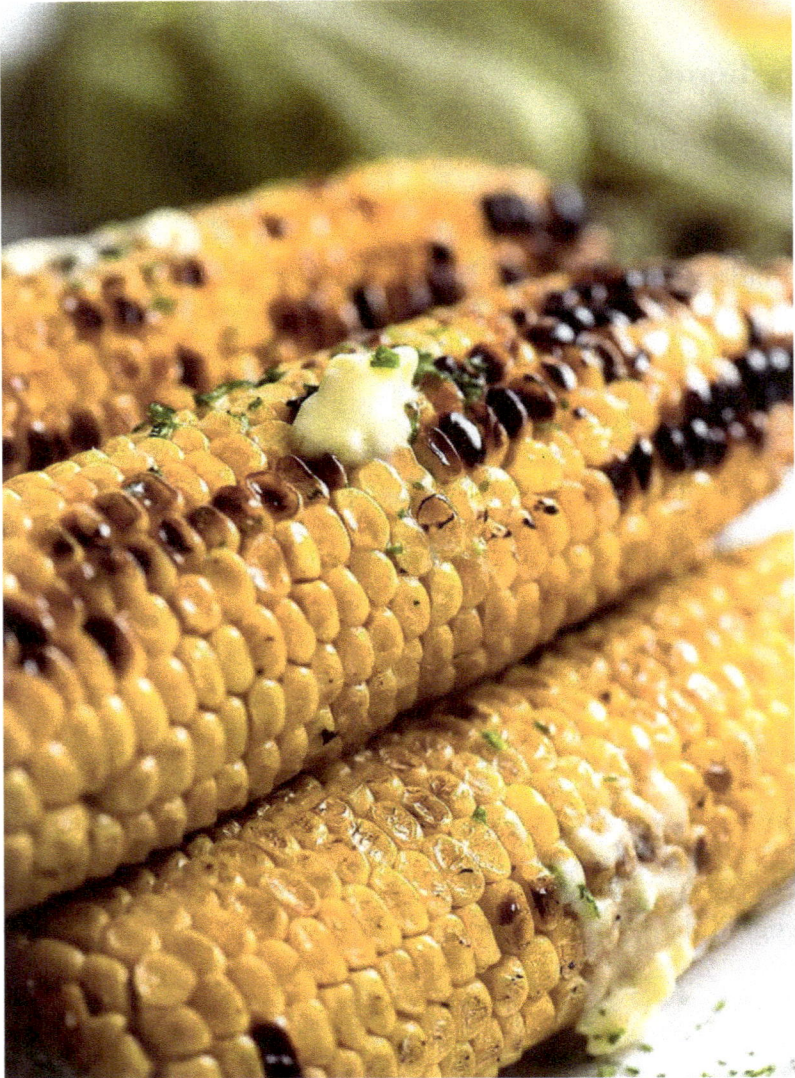

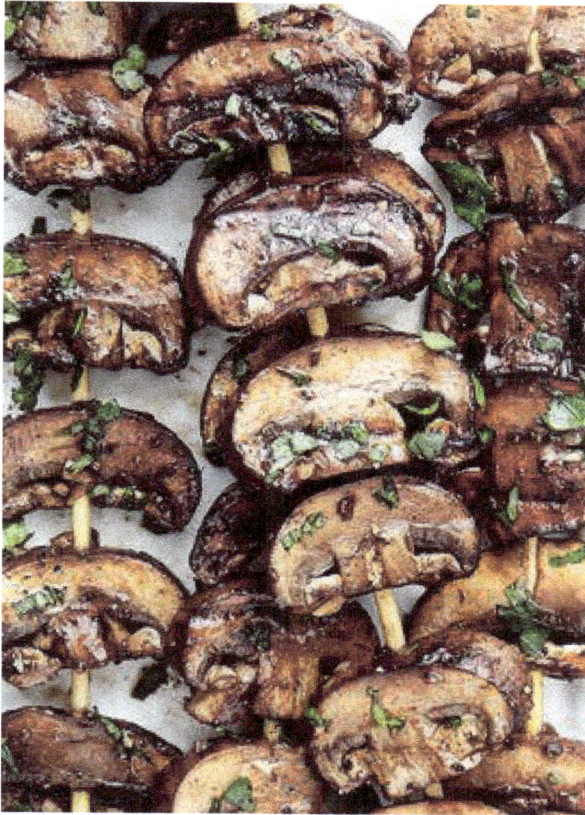

Ingredients

- 2 Corns, cut lengthwise

- 10 Crimini Mushrooms, rinsed and drained

Marinade Ingredients:

- 6 tbsp. extra virgin olive oil

- Sea salt, to taste

- 3 tbsp. distilled white vinegar

- 1 tsp. Dijon mustard

Directions:

Marinate the vegetable with the dressing or marinade ingredients for 15 to 30 min. Grill for 4 minutes over medium heat or until the vegetable becomes tender.

Grilled Zucchini and Pineapple

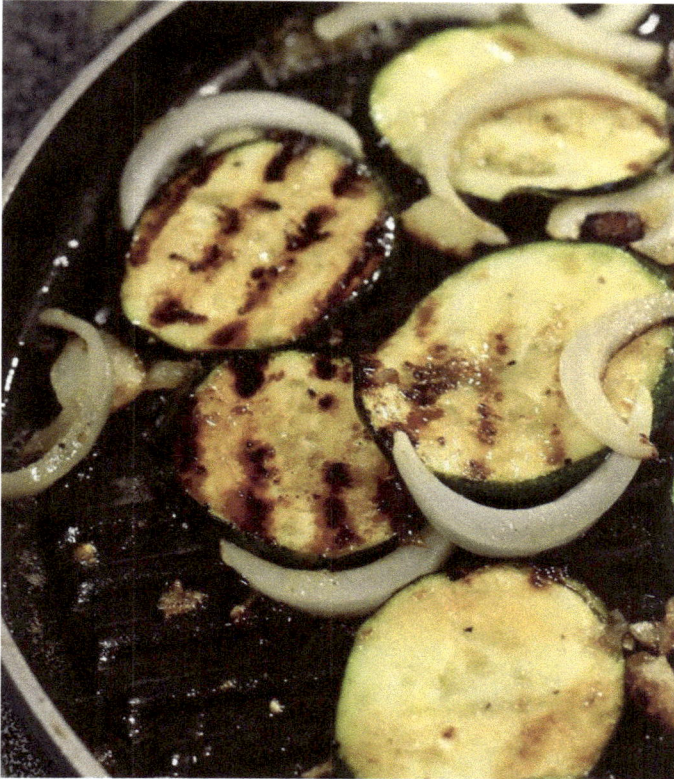

Ingredients

- 2 large zucchini , cut lengthwise into ½ inch slabs

- 2 large red onions, cut into ½ inch rings but don't separate into individual rings

- 1 medium Pineapple, cut into 1/2 inch slices

- 10 Green Beans

Marinade Ingredients:

- 6 tbsp. extra virgin olive oil

- Sea salt, to taste

- 3 tbsp. distilled white vinegar

- 1 tsp. honey

Directions:

Marinate the vegetable with the dressing or marinade ingredients for 15 to 30 min. Grill for 4 minutes over medium heat or until the vegetable becomes tender.

Grilled Asparagus and Mushrooms

Ingredients

- 6 pcs. Crimini mushrooms, rinsed and drained
- 2 pcs. Eggplant, cut lengthwise and cut in half
- 2 pcs. Zucchini, cut lengthwise and cut in half
- 6 pcs. Asparagus

<u>Dressing Ingredients</u>

- 6 tbsp. extra virgin olive oil
- Sea salt, to taste
- 3 tbsp. apple cider vinegar
  1 tbsp. honey
- 1 tsp. Egg-free mayonnaise

Directions:

Marinate the vegetable with the dressing or marinade ingredients for 15 to 30 min. Grill for 4 minutes over medium heat or until the vegetable becomes tender

Grilled Japanese Eggplant Bell Peppers and Broccolini

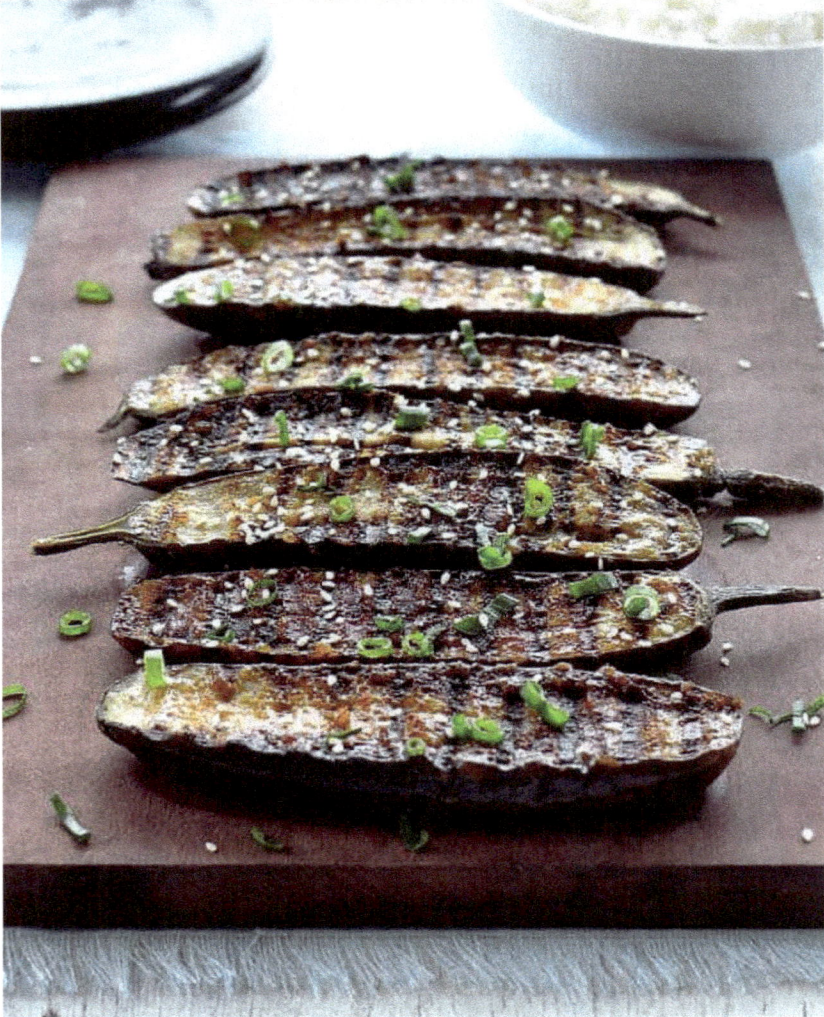

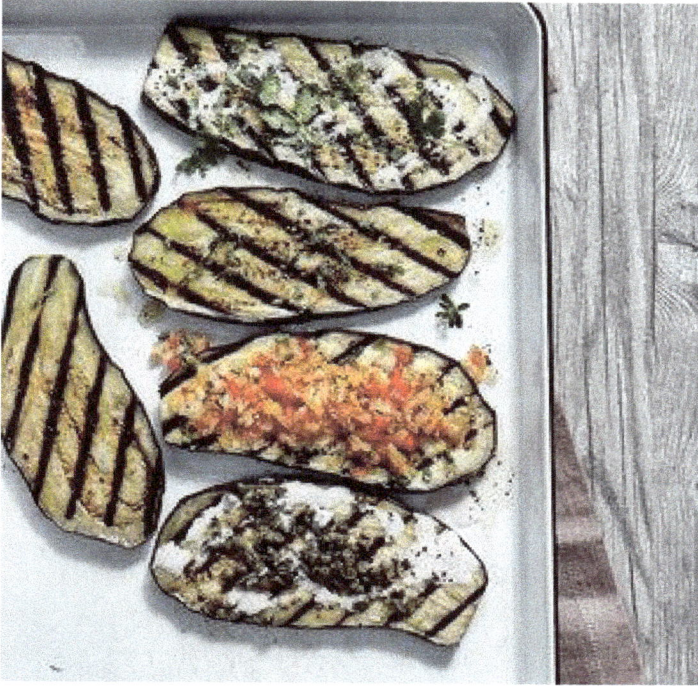

Ingredients

- 2 green Bell Peppers, cut in half

- 10 Broccolini Florets

- 2 pcs. Japanese Eggplant, cut lengthwise and cut in half

Dressing Ingredients

- 6 tbsp. sesame oil

- Sea salt, to taste

- 3 tbsp. distilled white vinegar

- 1 tsp. mayonnaise

Directions:

Marinate the vegetable with the dressing or marinade ingredients for 15 to 30 min. Grill for 4 minutes over medium heat or until the vegetable becomes tender.

Grilled Japanese Bell Pepper and Cauliflower Recipe with Balsamic Glaze

Ingredients

- 2 Yellow Bell Peppers, cut in half lengthwise

- 10 Cauliflower Florets

- 2 pcs. Japanese Eggplant, cut lengthwise and cut in half

Dressing Ingredients

- 6 tbsp. extra virgin olive oil

- Sea salt, to taste

- 3 tbsp. Balsamic vinegar

- 1 tsp. Dijon mustard

Directions:

Marinate the vegetable with the dressing or marinade ingredients for 15 to 30 min. Grill for 4 minutes over medium heat or until the vegetable becomes tender. Grilled Broccoli and Zucchini Recipe Ingredients 2 large Eggplants, cut lengthwise and cut in half 1 large Zucchini, cut lengthwise and cut in half 5

Grilled Eggplant and Yellow Bell Peppers

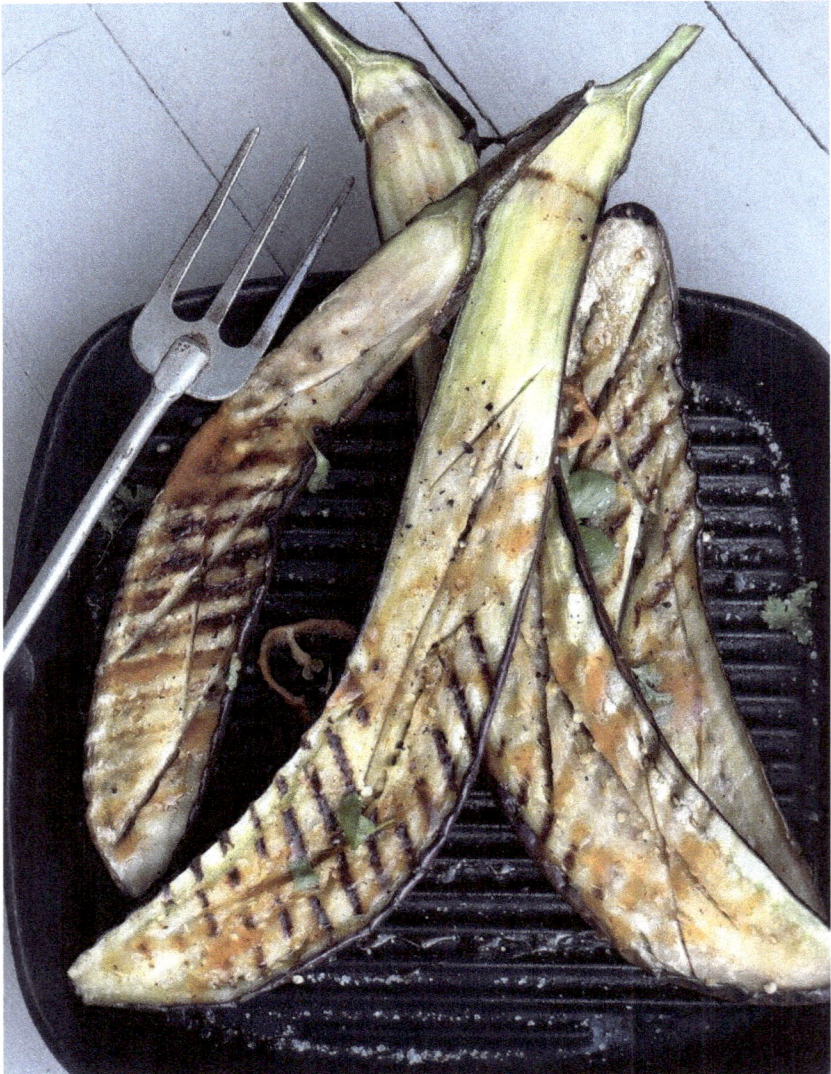

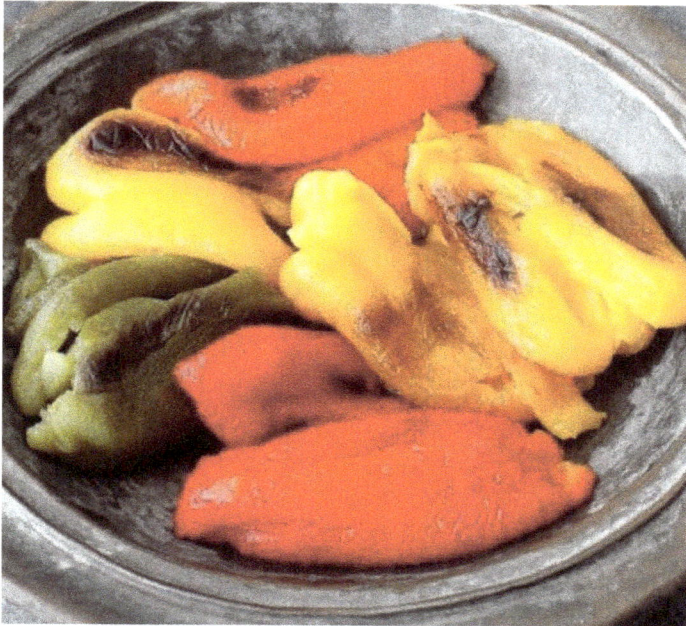

Ingredients

- 2 Yellow Bell Peppers, cut in half

- 10 Broccolini Florets

- 2 pcs. Eggplant, cut lengthwise and cut in half

Dressing Ingredients

- 6 tbsp. olive oil

- Sea salt, to taste

- 3 tbsp. white wine vinegar

- 1 tsp. mustard

Directions:

Marinate the vegetable with the dressing or marinade ingredients for 15 to 30 min. Grill for 4 minutes over medium heat or until the vegetable becomes tender.

Grilled Collard Greens and Portobello Mushrooms

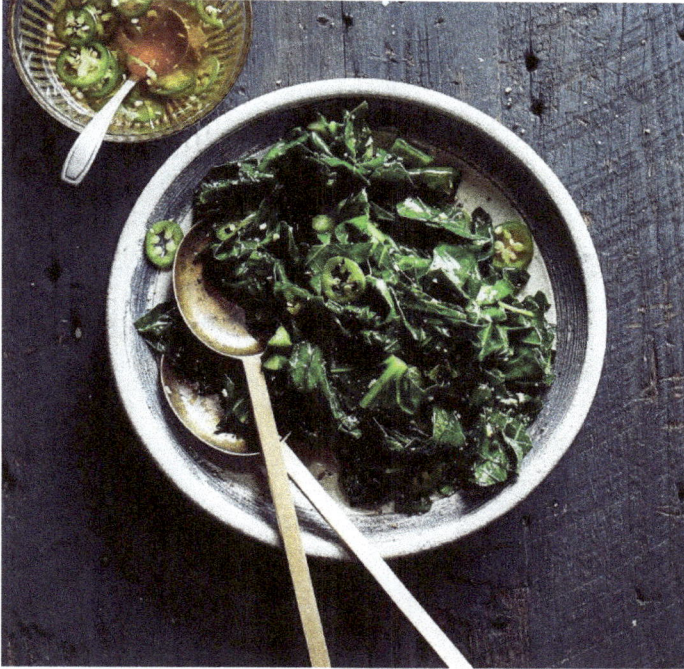

Ingredients

- 1 bunch of collard greens

- 5 pcs. Portobello mushrooms, rinsed and drained

- 10 Asparagus spears

Dressing Ingredients

- 6 tbsp. olive oil

- Sea salt, to taste

- 3 tbsp. white wine vinegar

- 1 tsp. Egg-free mayonnaise

Directions:

Marinate the vegetable with the dressing or marinade ingredients for 15 to 30 min. Grill for 4 minutes over medium heat or until the vegetable becomes tender.

Red Cabbage and Onion in Ranch Dressing

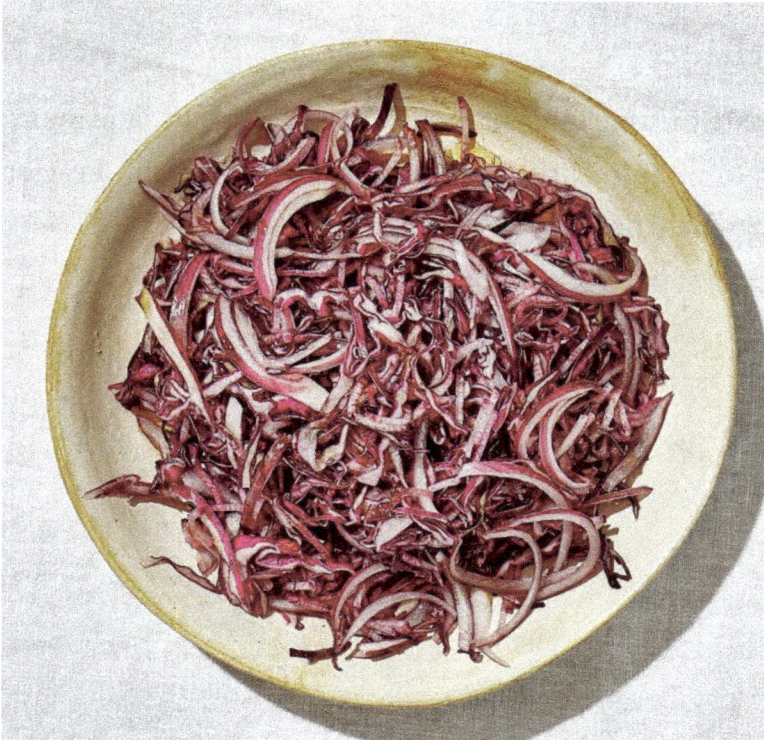

Ingredients

- 1 red cabbage
- 2 large red onions, cut into ½ inch rings but don't separate into individual rings
- 2 tbsp. extra virgin olive oil

- 2 tbsp. ranch dressing mix

Directions:

Marinate the vegetable with the dressing or marinade ingredients for 15 to 30 min. Grill for 4 minutes over medium heat or until the vegetable becomes tender.

Grilled Broccolini Asparagus and Eggplants

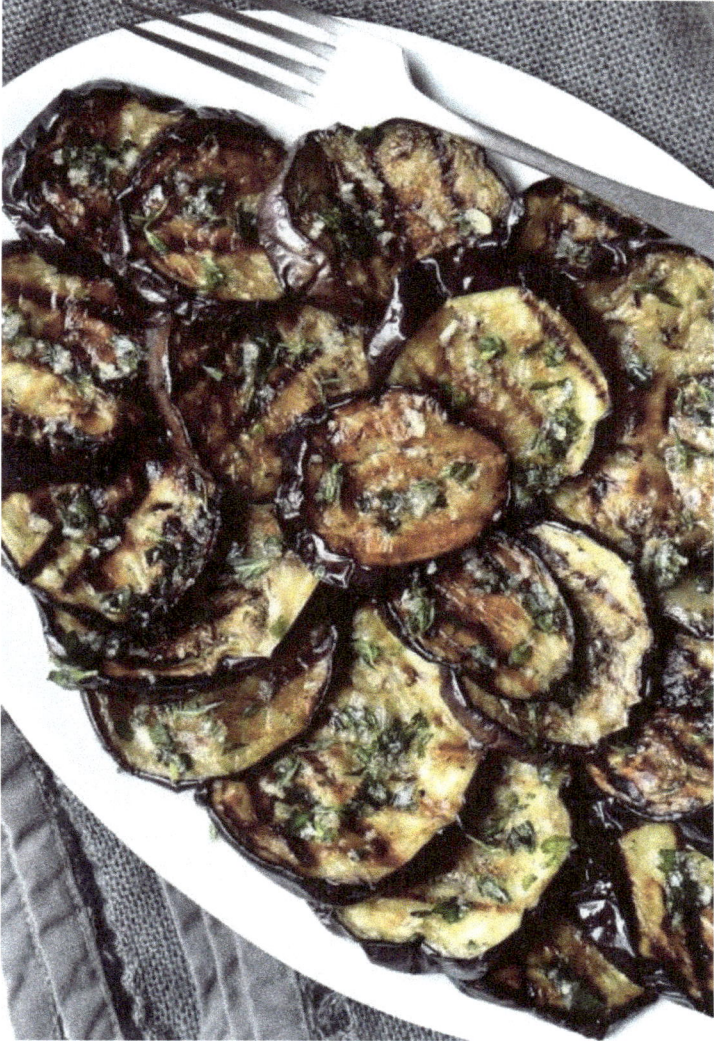

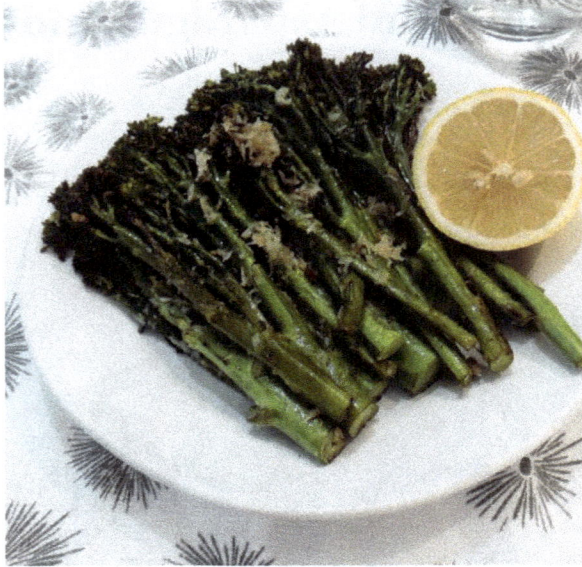

Ingredients

- 1 large Eggplants, cut lengthwise and cut in half
- 1 bunch of turnip greens
- 10 Asparagus spears
- 10 Broccolini Florets

Marinade Ingredients:

- 6 tbsp. extra virgin olive oil
- Sea salt, to taste 3 tbsp.

- distilled white vinegar

- 1 tsp. Dijon mustard

Directions:

Marinate the vegetable with the dressing or marinade ingredients for 15 to 30 min. Grill for 4 minutes over medium heat or until the vegetable becomes tender.

Grilled Rutabaga and Mustard Greens

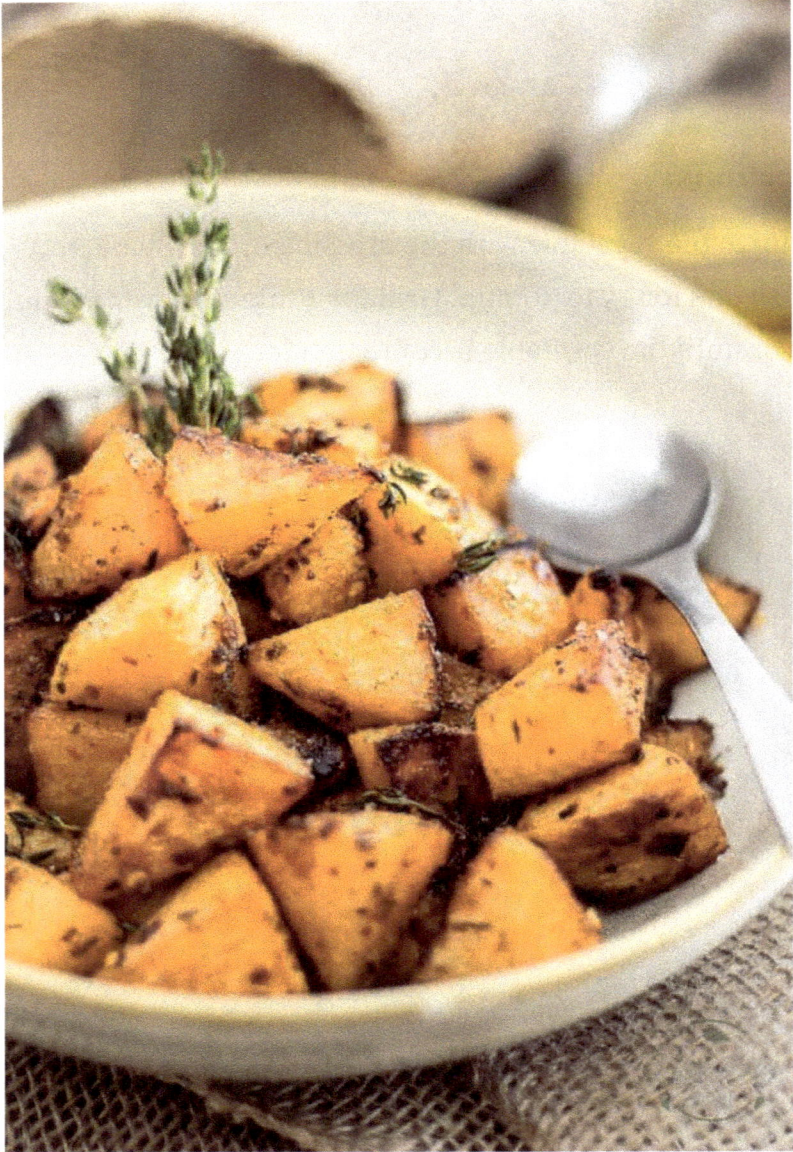

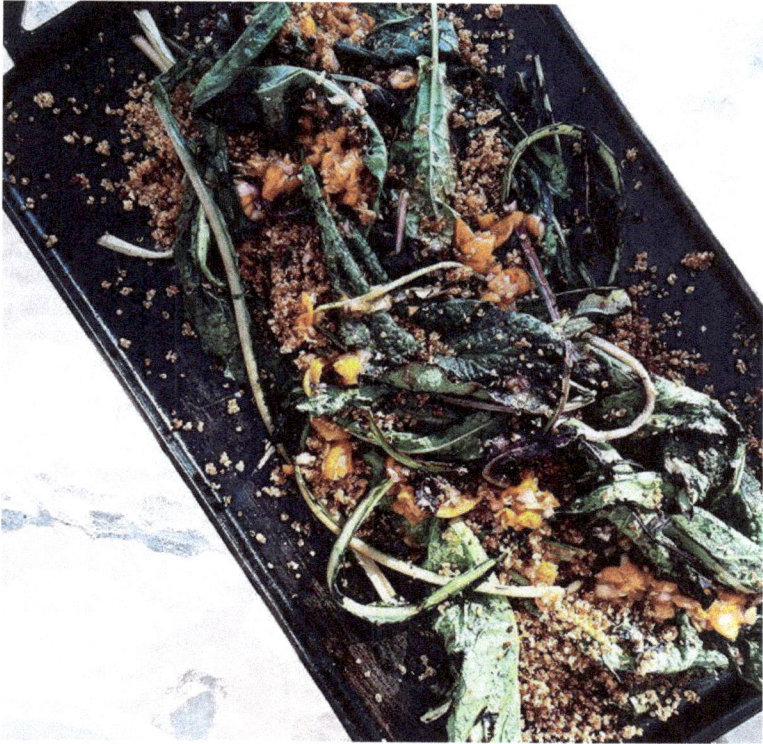

Ingredients

- 1 medium Rutabaga, peeled and cut in half lengthwise

- 1 large red onion, cut into ½ inch rings but don't separate into individual rings

- 1 bunch of mustard greens

Dressing Ingredients

- 6 tbsp. olive oil

- Sea salt, to taste

- 3 tbsp. white wine vinegar

- 1 tsp. English mustard

Directions:

Marinate the vegetable with the dressing or marinade ingredients for 15 to 30 min. Grill for 4 minutes over medium heat or until the vegetable becomes tender.

Grilled Turnips with Broccoli

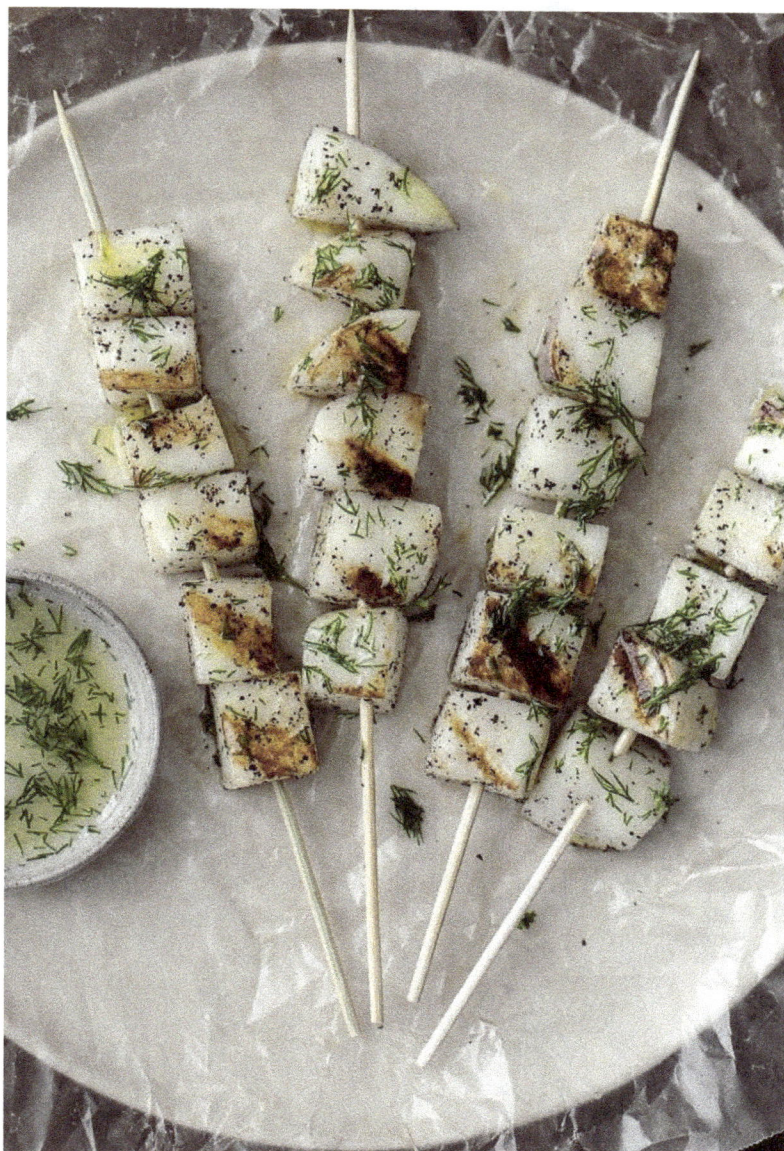

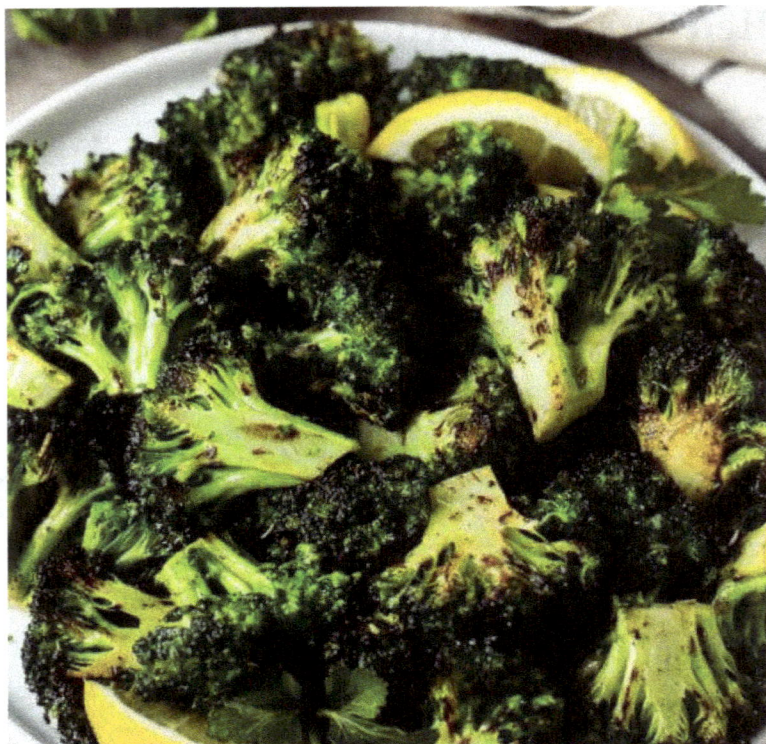

Ingredients

- 10 Broccoli florets

- 1 large turnips, peeled and cut lengthwise

- 1 red cabbage, cut in half

Dressing Ingredients

- 6 tbsp. olive oil

- Sea salt, to taste

- 3 tbsp. white wine vinegar

- 1 tsp. Egg-free mayonnaise

Directions:

Marinate the vegetable with the dressing or marinade ingredients for 15 to 30 min. Grill for 4 minutes over medium heat or until the vegetable becomes tender.

Grilled Turnip and Beetroots

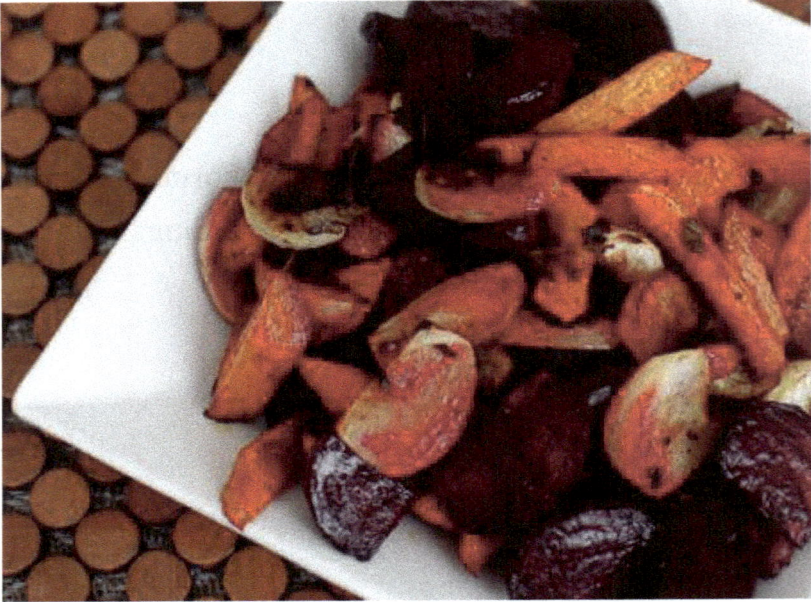

Ingredients

- 1 large turnip, peeled and cut lengthwise

- 1 large carrot, peeled and cut lengthwise

- 1 medium Beetroot, peeled and cut in half lengthwise

Dressing Ingredients

- 6 tbsp. sesame oil

- Sea salt, to taste

- 3 tbsp. distilled white vinegar

- 1 tsp. Egg-free mayonnaise

Directions:

Marinate the vegetable with the dressing or marinade ingredients for 15 to 30 min. Grill for 4 minutes over medium heat or until the vegetable becomes tender.

Grilled Water Chestnuts and Mangoes

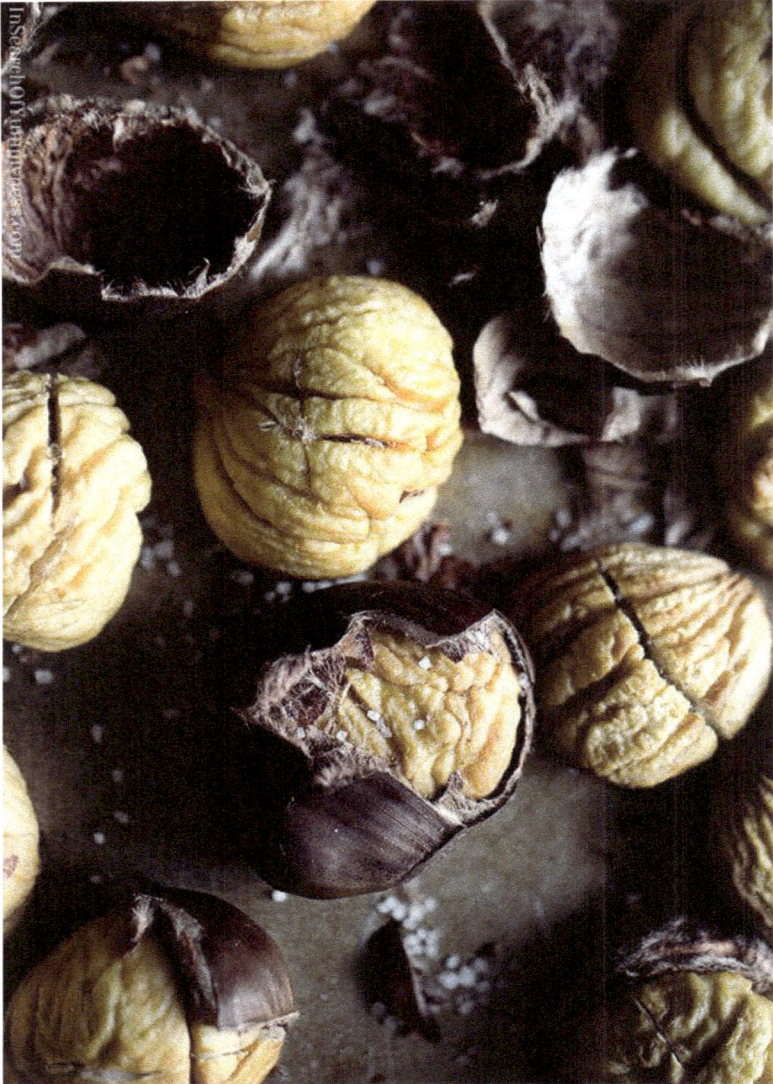

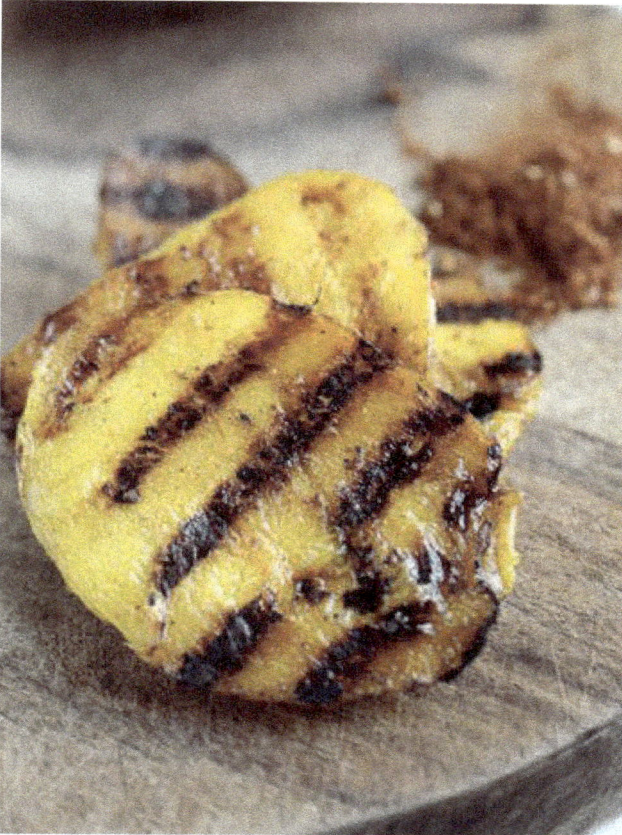

Ingredients

- 1/2 cup water chestnuts

- 2 large mangoes, cut lengthwise and pitted

Dressing Ingredients

- 6 tbsp. sesame oil

- Sea salt, to taste

- 3 tbsp. distilled white vinegar

- 1 tsp. Egg-free mayonnaise

Directions:

Marinate the vegetable with the dressing or marinade ingredients for 15 to 30 min. Grill for 4 minutes over medium heat or until the vegetable becomes tender. For the mango, grill only until you start seeing brown grill marks.

Grilled Artichoke Hearts and Water Chestnuts

Ingredients

- ½ cup canned artichoke hearts

- 1/2 cup water chestnuts

- 10 pcs. Brussel Sprouts

Dressing Ingredients

- 6 tbsp. olive oil

- Sea salt, to taste

- 3 tbsp. white wine vinegar

- 1 tsp. Egg-free mayonnaise

Directions:

Marinate the vegetable with the dressing or marinade ingredients for 15 to 30 min. Grill for 4 minutes over medium heat or until the vegetable becomes tender.

Grilled Assorted Bell Peppers with Broccolini Florets Recipe

Ingredients

- 1 Green Bell Pepper, cut in half
- 2 beetroots, peeled and sliced lengthwise
- 1 red Bell Pepper, cut in half
- 10 Broccolini Florets

Marinade Ingredients:

- 6 tbsp. extra virgin olive oil
- Sea salt, to taste
- 3 tbsp. distilled white vinegar
- 1 tsp. Dijon mustard

Directions:

Marinate the vegetable with the dressing or marinade ingredients for 15 to 30 min. Grill for 4 minutes over medium heat or until the vegetable becomes tender.

Grilled Portobello and Rutabaga

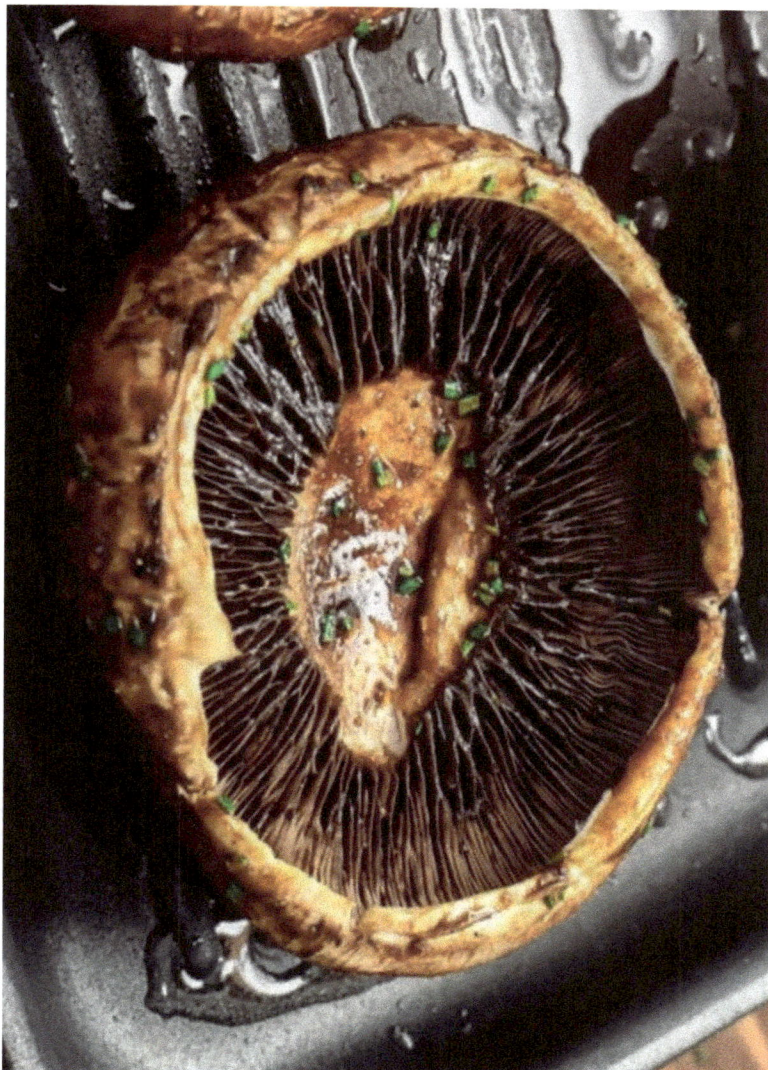

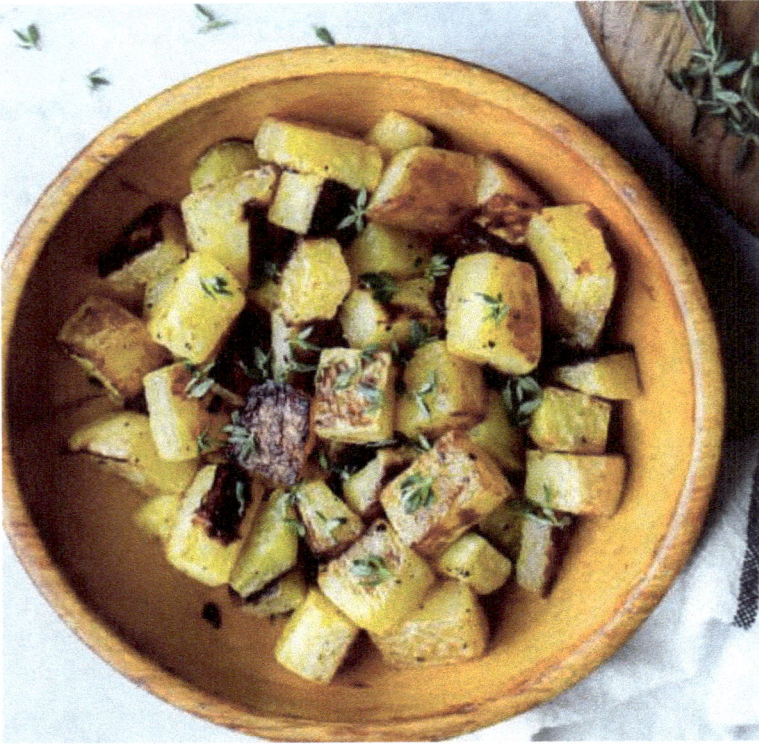

Ingredients

- 1 medium Rutabaga, peeled and cut in half lengthwise

- 5 pcs. Portobello mushrooms, rinsed and drained

- 1 medium red onion, cut into ½ inch rings but don't separate into individual rings

Dressing Ingredients

- 6 tbsp. extra virgin olive oil

- Sea salt, to taste

- 3 tbsp. Balsamic vinegar

- 1 tsp. Dijon mustard

Directions:

Marinate the vegetable with the dressing or marinade ingredients for 15 to 30 min. Grill for 4 minutes over medium heat or until the vegetable becomes tender.

Grilled Brussel Sprouts Cauliflower and Rutabaga

Ingredients

- 1 medium Rutabaga, peeled and cut in half lengthwise

- 10 Cauliflower florets

- 5 pcs. Brussel Sprouts

- 1 bunch of collard greens

<u>Dressing Ingredients</u>

- 6 tbsp. olive oil

- Sea salt, to taste

- 3 tbsp. white wine vinegar

- 1 tsp. English mustard

Directions:

Marinate the vegetable with the dressing or marinade ingredients for 15 to 30 min. Grill for 4 minutes over medium heat or until the vegetable becomes tender.

Grilled Water Chestnuts Swiss Chard and Asparagus Recipe

Ingredients

- 1/2 cup water chestnuts

- 1 bunch of swiss chard

- 6 pcs. Asparagus

- Dressing Ingredients

- 6 tbsp. extra virgin olive oil

- Sea salt, to taste

- 3 tbsp. apple cider vinegar

- 1 tbsp. honey

- 1 tsp. Egg-free mayonnaise

Directions:

Marinate the vegetable with the dressing or marinade ingredients for 15 to 30 min. Grill for 4 minutes over medium heat or until the vegetable becomes tender.

Grilled Asparagus Pineapple and Green Beans

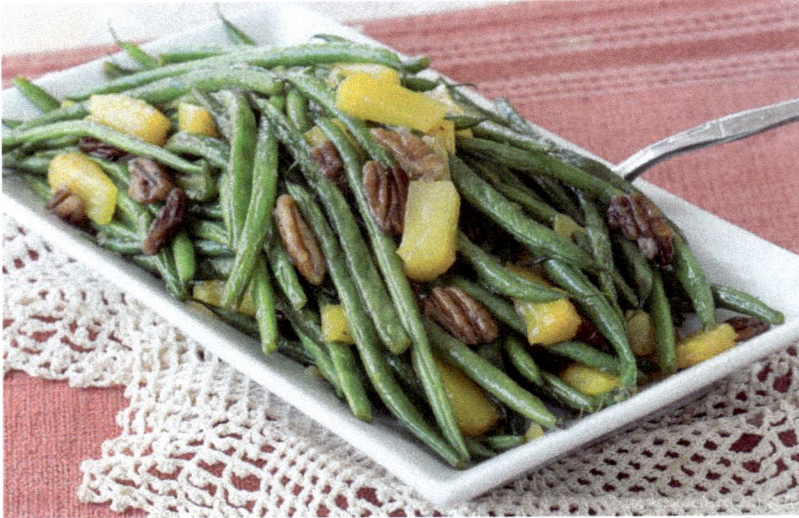

Ingredients

- 1 medium Rutabaga, peeled and cut in half lengthwise

- 10 pcs. Asparagus

- 1 medium Pineapple, cut into 1/2 inch slices

- 1 bunch of collard greens

Dressing Ingredients

- 6 tbsp. sesame oil

- Sea salt, to taste

- 3 tbsp. distilled white vinegar

- 1 tsp. Egg-free mayonnaise

Directions:

Marinate the vegetable with the dressing or marinade ingredients for 15 to 30 min. Grill for 4 minutes over medium heat or until the vegetable becomes tender.

Asparagus Dressing

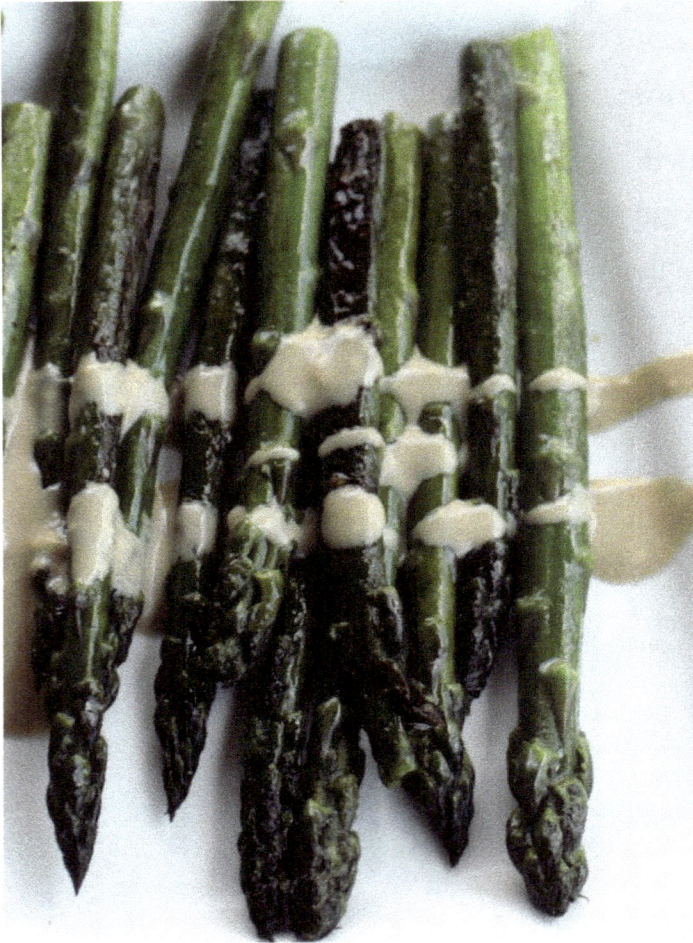

Ingredients

- 6 tbsp. sesame oil

- Sea salt, to taste

- 3 tbsp. distilled white vinegar

- 1 tsp. Egg-free mayonnaise

Directions:

Marinate the vegetable with the dressing or marinade ingredients for 15 to 30 min. Grill for 4 minutes over medium heat or until the vegetable becomes tender.

Grilled Broccoli & Swiss Chard

Ingredients

- 2 green Bell Peppers, cut in half

- 1 bunch of swiss chard

- 5 Broccoli Florets Dressing Ingredients

- 6 tbsp. sesame oil

- Sea salt, to taste

- 3 tbsp. distilled white vinegar

- 1 tsp. Egg-free mayonnaise

Directions:

Marinate the vegetable with the dressing or marinade ingredients for 15 to 30 min. Grill for 4 minutes over medium heat or until the vegetable becomes tender.

Grilled Water Chestnuts and Green Beans

Ingredients

- 10 Broccolini Florets

- 10 pcs. Asparagus

- 1/2 cup water chestnuts

- 10 Green Beans

- <u>Marinade Ingredients:</u>

- 6 tbsp. extra virgin olive oil

- Sea salt, to taste

- 3 tbsp. distilled white vinegar

- 1 tsp. Dijon mustard

Directions:

Marinate the vegetable with the dressing or marinade ingredients for 15 to 30 min. Grill for 4 minutes over medium heat or until the vegetable becomes tender.

Grilled Turnip Greens and Okra

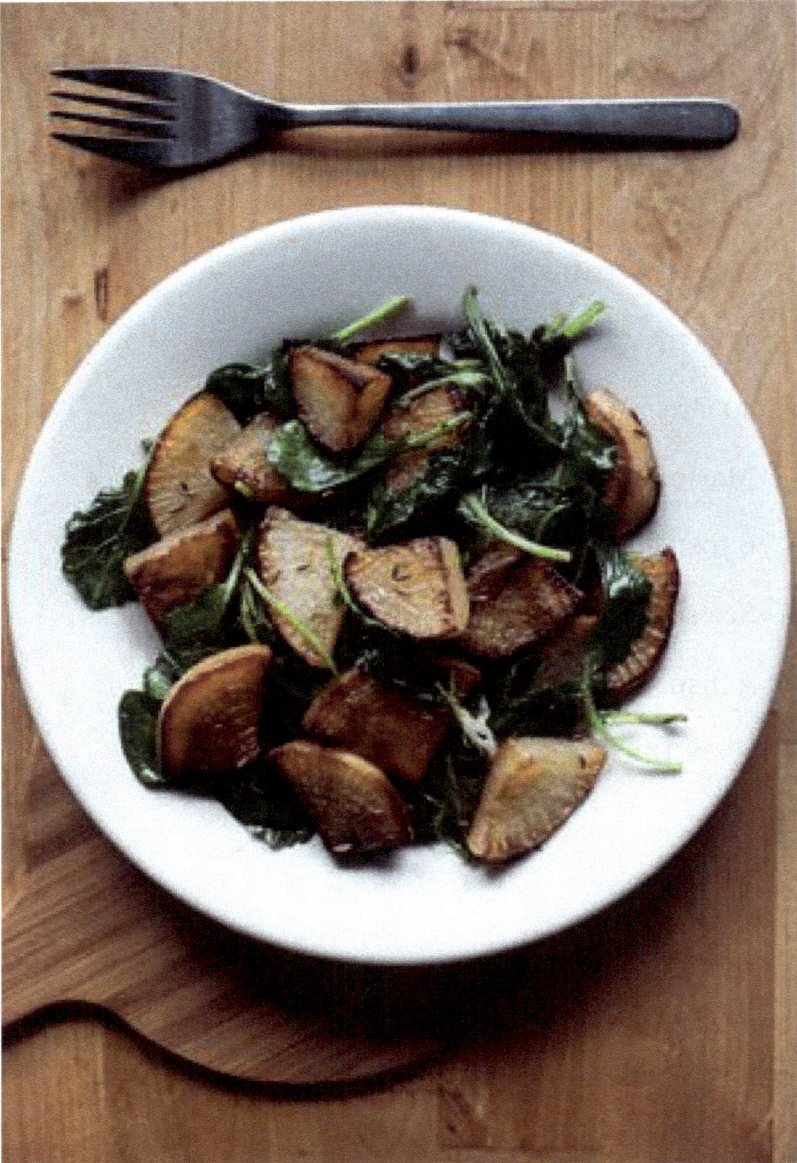

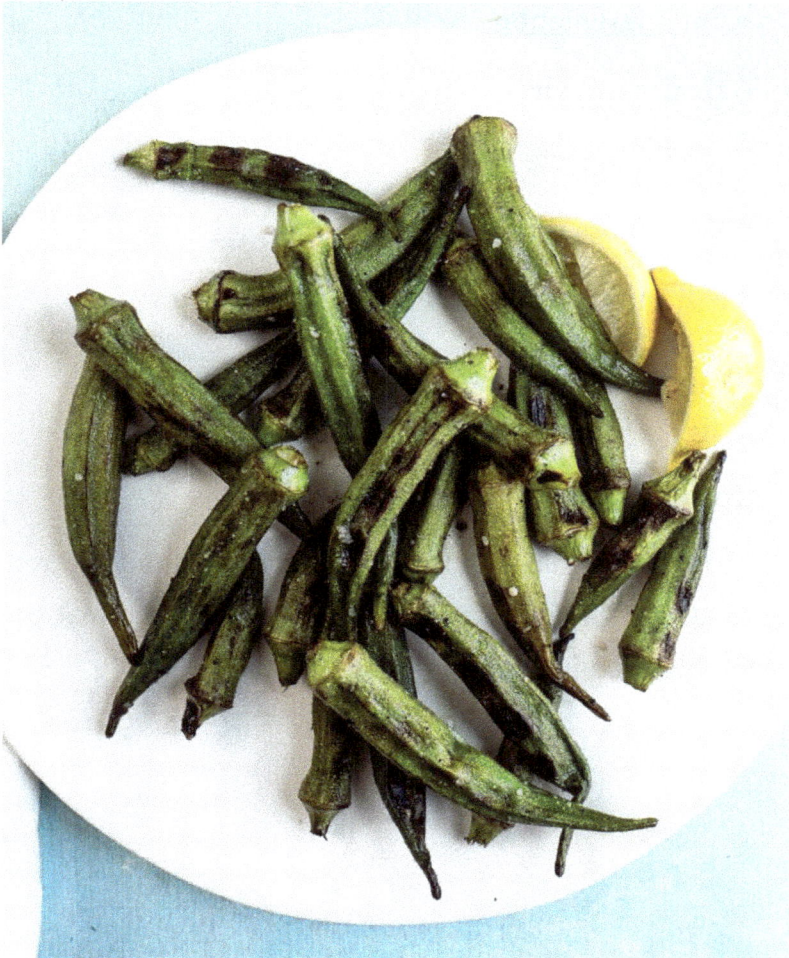

Ingredients

- 5 pcs. Okra

- 1 bunch of turnip greens

- 2 large red onions, cut into ½ inch rings but don't separate into individual rings

Dressing Ingredients

- 6 tbsp. extra virgin olive oil

- Sea salt, to taste

- 3 tbsp. Balsamic vinegar

- 1 tsp. Dijon mustard

Directions:

Marinate the vegetable with the dressing or marinade ingredients for 15 to 30 min. Grill for 4 minutes over medium heat or until the vegetable becomes tender.

Grilled Beetroots and Purple Cabbage

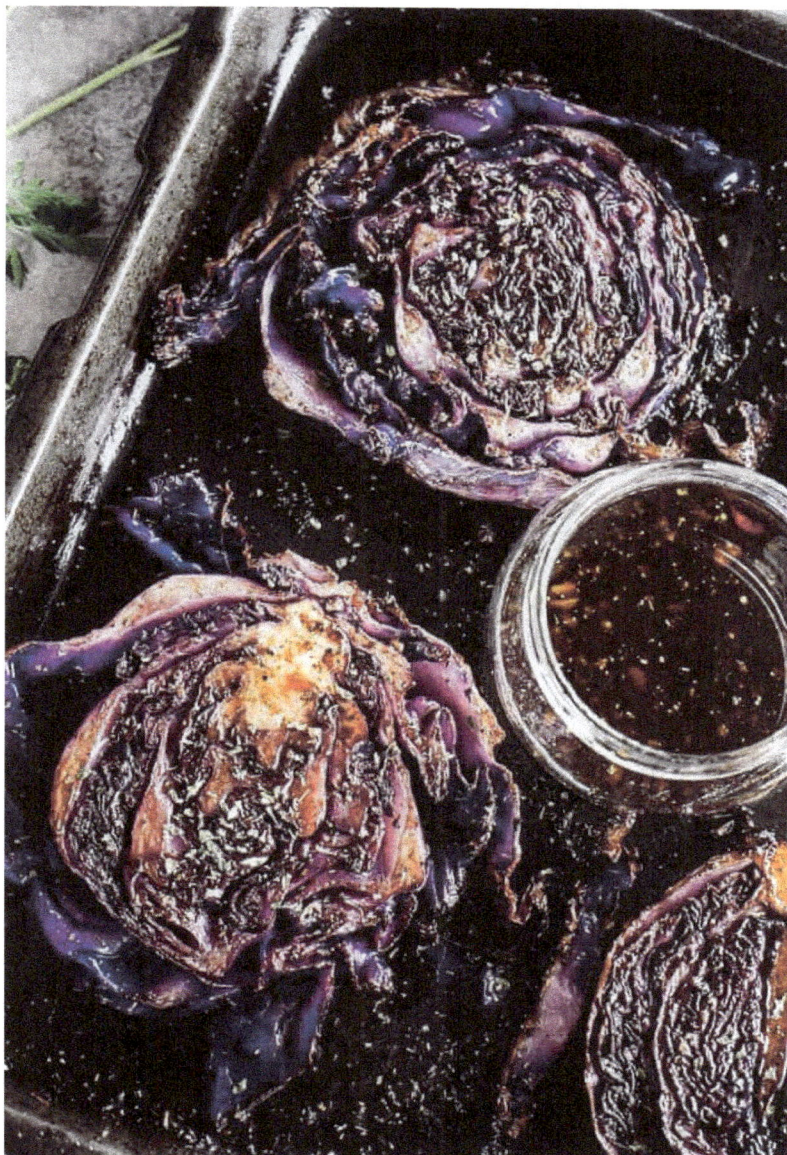

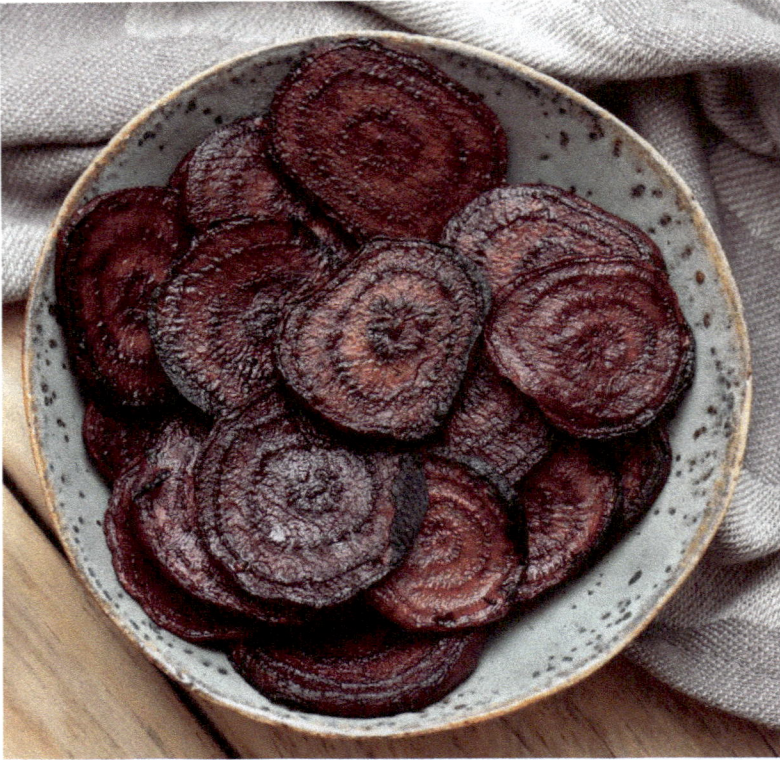

Ingredients

- 1 large Parsnip, cut lengthwise

- 1 Purple cabbage

- 2 beetroots, peeled and sliced lengthwise

- 2 large Zucchinis, cut lengthwise and cut in half

Dressing Ingredients

- 6 tbsp. olive oil

- Sea salt, to taste

- 3 tbsp. white wine vinegar

- 1 tsp. English mustard

Directions:

Marinate the vegetable with the dressing or marinade ingredients for 15 to 30 min. Grill for 4 minutes over medium heat or until the vegetable becomes tender.

Grilled Turnip and Endives

Ingredients

- 1 large Turnip, cut lengthwise
- 2 green Bell Peppers, cut in half
- 1 bunch of endives
- Dressing Ingredients
- 6 tbsp. extra virgin olive oil
- Sea salt, to taste
- 3 tbsp. apple cider vinegar
- 1 tbsp. honey
- 1 tsp. Egg-free mayonnaise

Directions:

Marinate the vegetable with the dressing or marinade ingredients for 15 to 30 min. Grill for 4 minutes over medium heat or until the vegetable becomes tender.

Grilled Green Beans and Pineapple

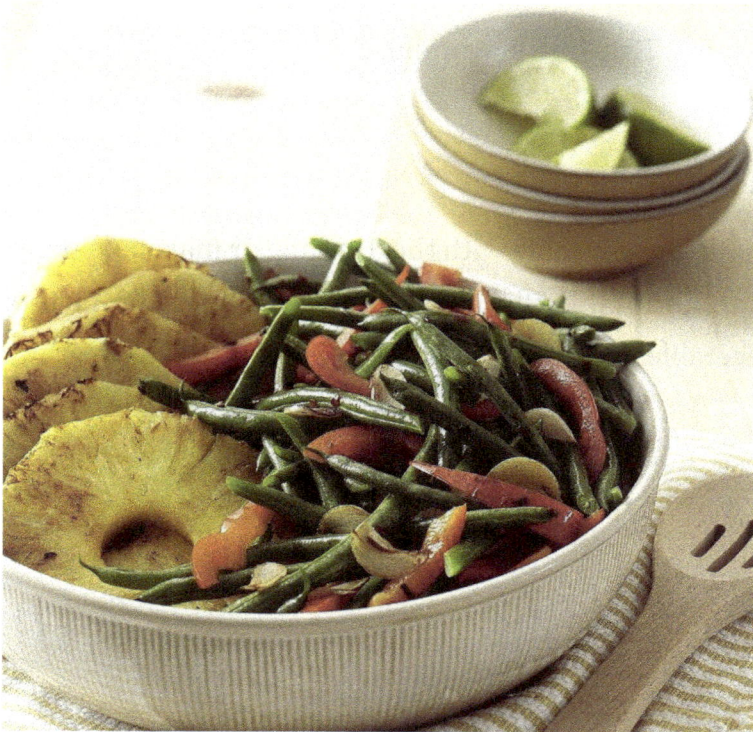

Ingredients

- 1 large Turnip, cut lengthwise

- 1 medium Pineapple, cut into 1/2 inch slices

- 10 Green Beans

Dressing Ingredients

- 6 tbsp. sesame oil

- Sea salt, to taste

- 3 tbsp. distilled white vinegar

- 1 tsp. Egg-free mayonnaise

Directions:

Marinate the vegetable with the dressing or marinade ingredients for 15 to 30 min. Grill for 4 minutes over medium heat or until the vegetable becomes tender.

Grilled Turnip and Zucchini

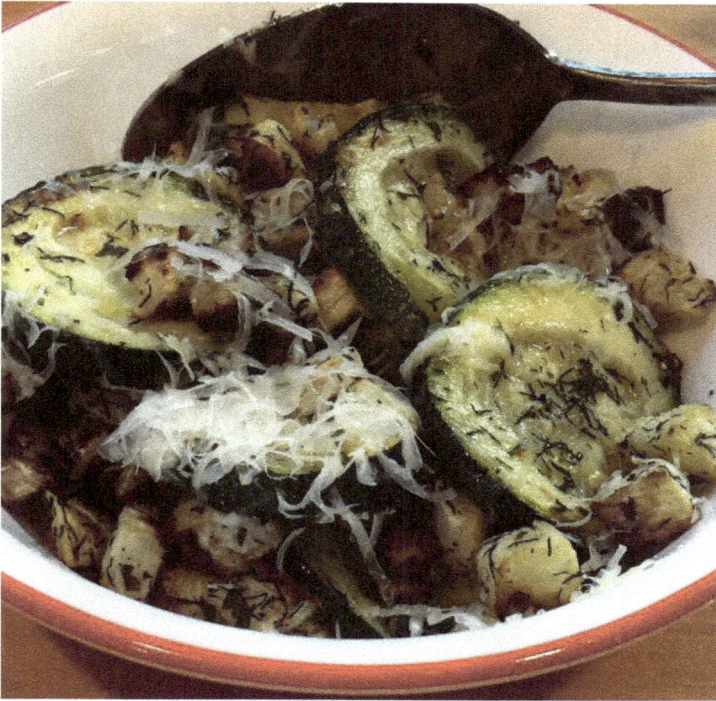

Ingredients

- 1 large Turnip, cut lengthwise

- 1 bunch of turnip greens

- 1 large zucchini , cut lengthwise into ½ inch slabs

- 2 small red onions, cut into ½ inch rings but don't separate into individual rings

Dressing Ingredients

- 6 tbsp. extra virgin olive oil

- Sea salt, to taste

- 3 tbsp. Balsamic vinegar

- 1 tsp. Dijon mustard

Directions:

Marinate the vegetable with the dressing or marinade ingredients for 15 to 30 min. Grill for 4 minutes over medium heat or until the vegetable becomes tender.

Grilled Portobello Mushrooms and Broccolini Florets

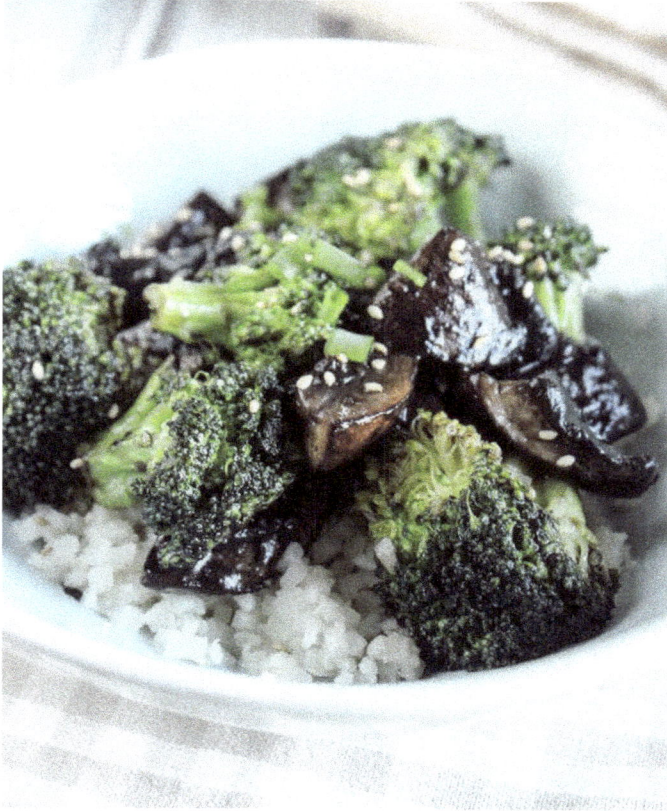

Ingredients

- 10 Broccolini Florets

- 10 pcs. Asparagus Corns, cut lengthwise

- 5 pcs. Portobello mushrooms, rinsed and drained

Marinade Ingredients:

- 6 tbsp. extra virgin olive oil

- Sea salt, to taste

- 3 tbsp. distilled white vinegar

- 1 tsp. Dijon mustard

Directions:

Marinate the vegetable with the dressing or marinade ingredients for 15 to 30 min. Grill for 4 minutes over medium heat or until the vegetable becomes tender.

Grilled Beetroots and Artichoke Hearts

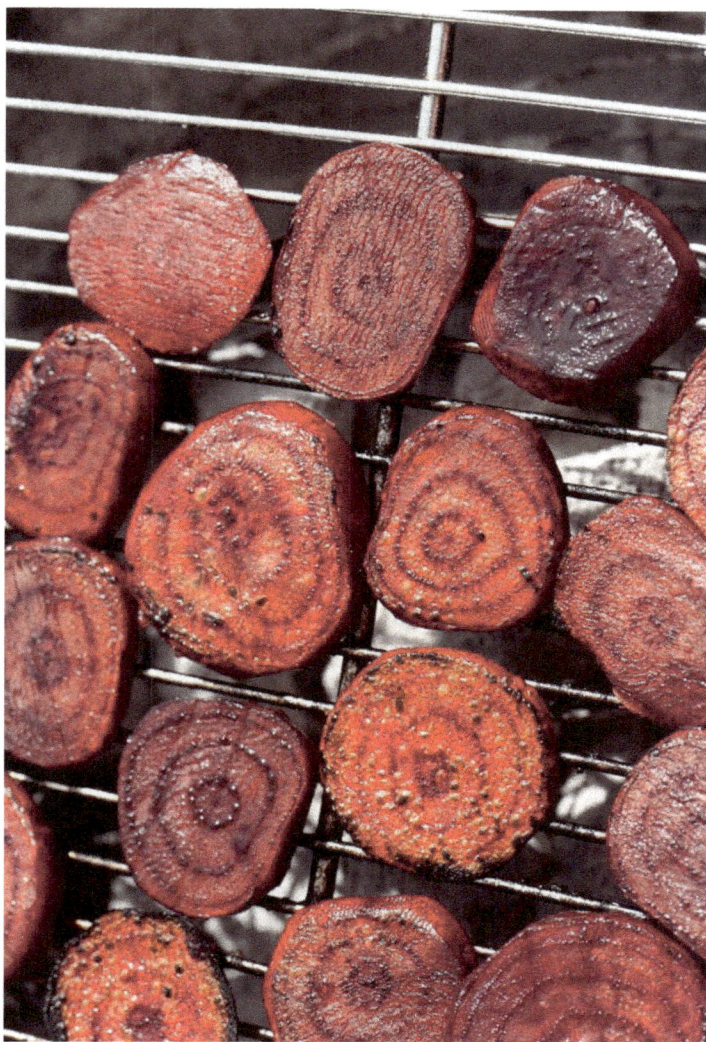

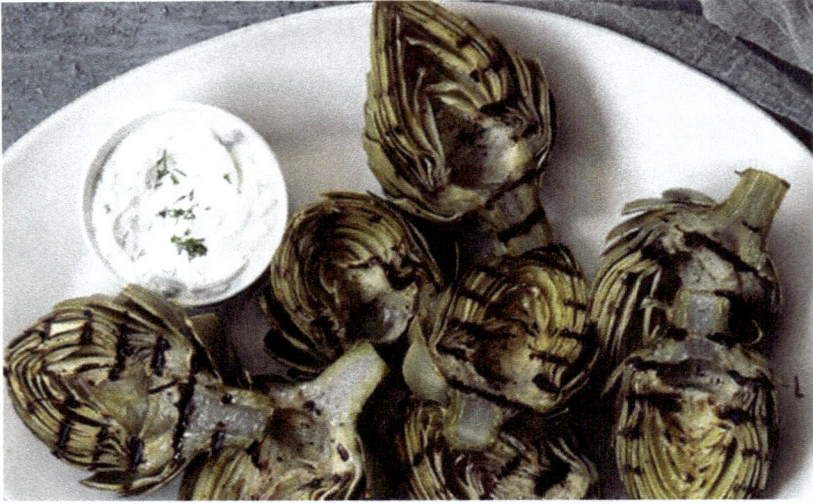

Ingredients

- ½ cup canned artichoke hearts

- 10 Broccolini Florets

- 2 beetroots, peeled and sliced lengthwise

Dressing Ingredients

- 6 tbsp. sesame oil

- Sea salt, to taste

- 3 tbsp. distilled white vinegar

- 1 tsp. Egg-free mayonnaise

Directions:

Marinate the vegetable with the dressing or marinade ingredients for 15 to 30 min. Grill for 4 minutes over medium heat or until the vegetable becomes tender.

Grilled Baby Carrots and Zucchini

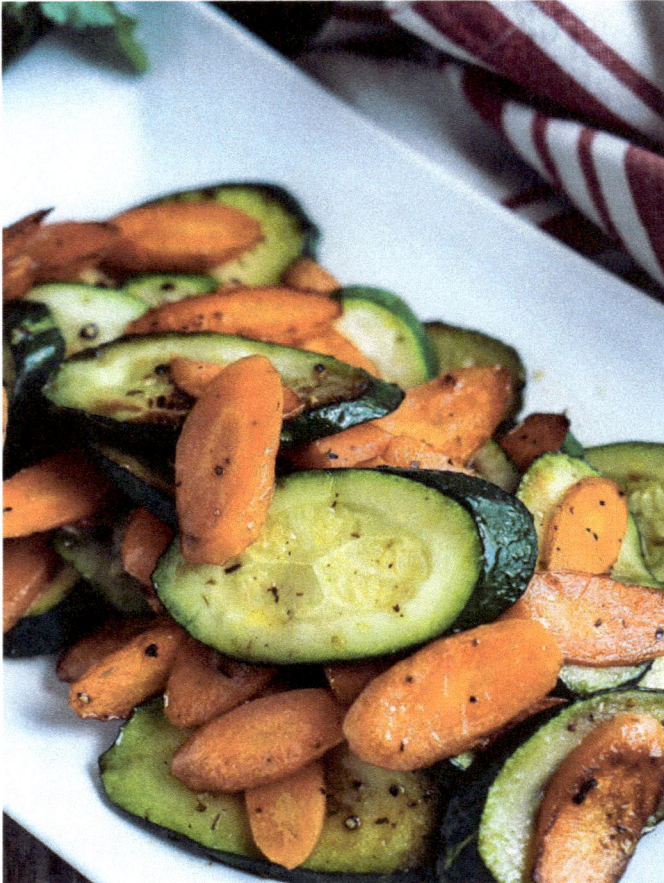

Ingredients

- 7 pcs. baby carrots
- 2 large zucchini, cut lengthwise into ½ inch slabs

- 2 large red onions, cut into ½ inch rings but don't separate into individual rings

Dressing Ingredients

- 6 tbsp. olive oil

- Sea salt, to taste

- 3 tbsp. white wine vinegar

- 1 tsp. Egg-free mayonnaise

Directions:

Marinate the vegetable with the dressing or marinade ingredients for 15 to 30 min. Grill for 4 minutes over medium heat or until the vegetable becomes tender.

Grilled Water Chestnuts Baby Carrots and Artichoke Hearts

Ingredients

- 1 cup canned artichoke hearts

- 1/2 cup canned water chestnuts

- 8 pcs. baby carrots

Dressing Ingredients

- 6 tbsp. olive oil

- Sea salt, to taste

- 3 bsp. white wine vinegar

- 1 tsp. English mustard

Directions:

Marinate the vegetable with the dressing or marinade ingredients for 15 to 30 min. Grill for 4 minutes over medium heat or until the vegetable becomes tender.

Grilled Rutabaga Zucchini and Onions

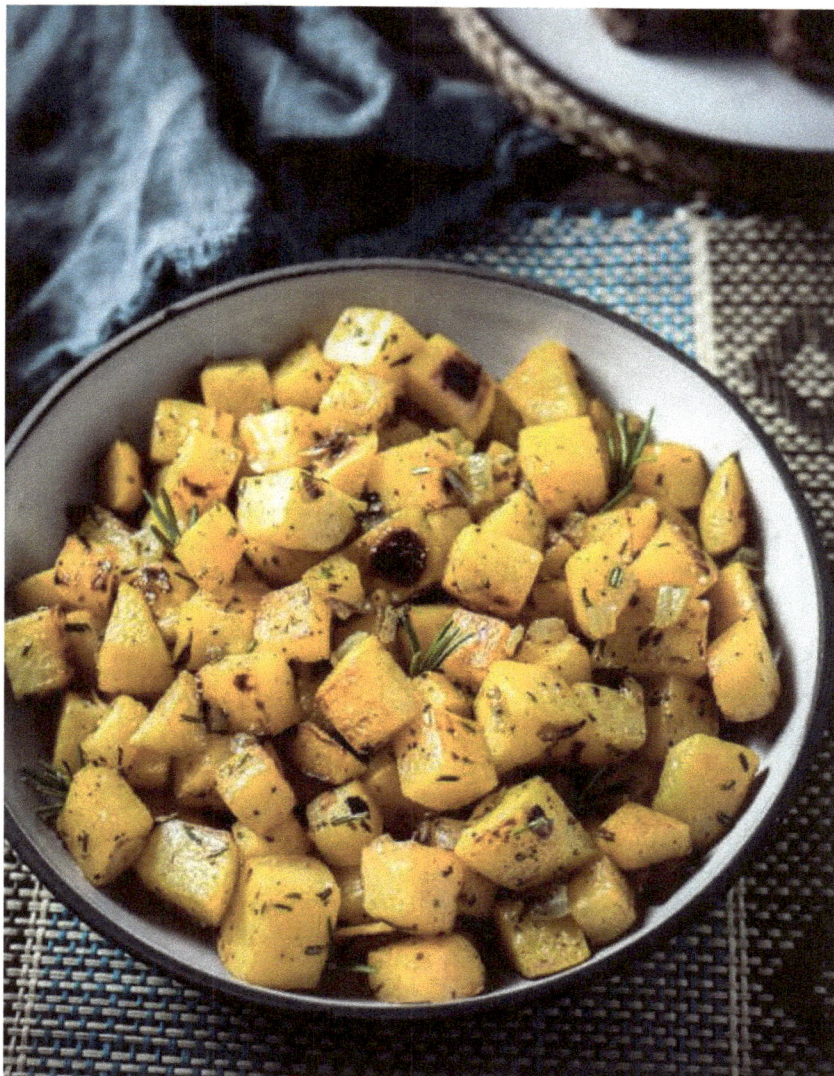

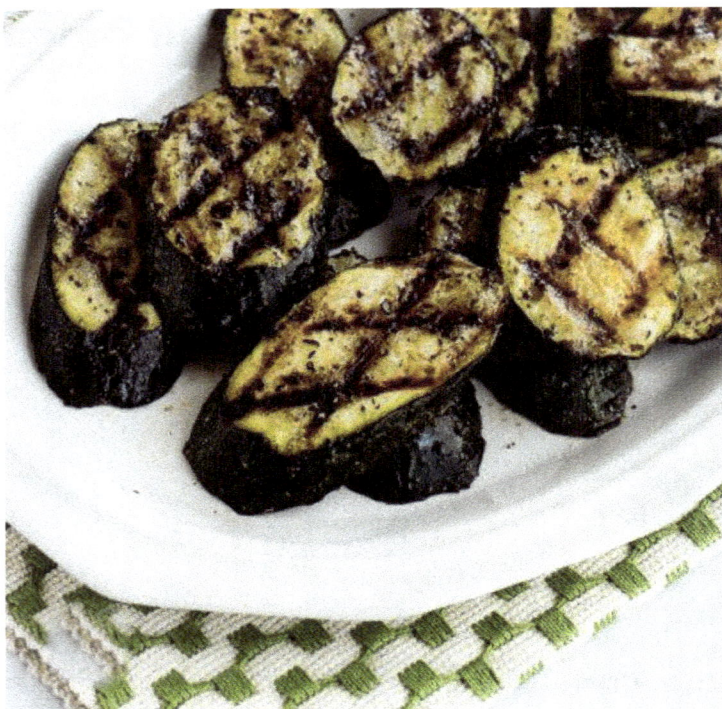

Ingredients

- 1 medium Rutabaga, peeled and cut in half lengthwise

- 2 large zucchini , cut lengthwise into ½ inch slabs

- 2 large red onions, cut into ½ inch rings but don't separate into individual rings

Dressing Ingredients

- 6 tbsp. olive oil

- Sea salt, to taste

- 3 tbsp. white wine vinegar

- 1 tsp. Egg-free mayonnaise

Directions:

Marinate the vegetable with the dressing or marinade ingredients for 15 to 30 min. Grill for 4 minutes over medium heat or until the vegetable becomes tender.

Grilled Rutabaga Broccolini Florets and Bell Peppers

Ingredients

- 1 medium Rutabaga, peeled and cut in half lengthwise

- 2 green Bell Peppers, cut in half

- 10 Broccolini Florets

Dressing Ingredients

- 6 tbsp. sesame oil

- Sea salt, to taste

- 3 tbsp. distilled white vinegar

- 1 tsp. Egg-free mayonnaise

Directions:

Marinate the vegetable with the dressing or marinade ingredients for 15 to 30 min. Grill for 4 minutes over medium heat or until the vegetable becomes tender.

Grilled Baby Carrots and Winter Squash

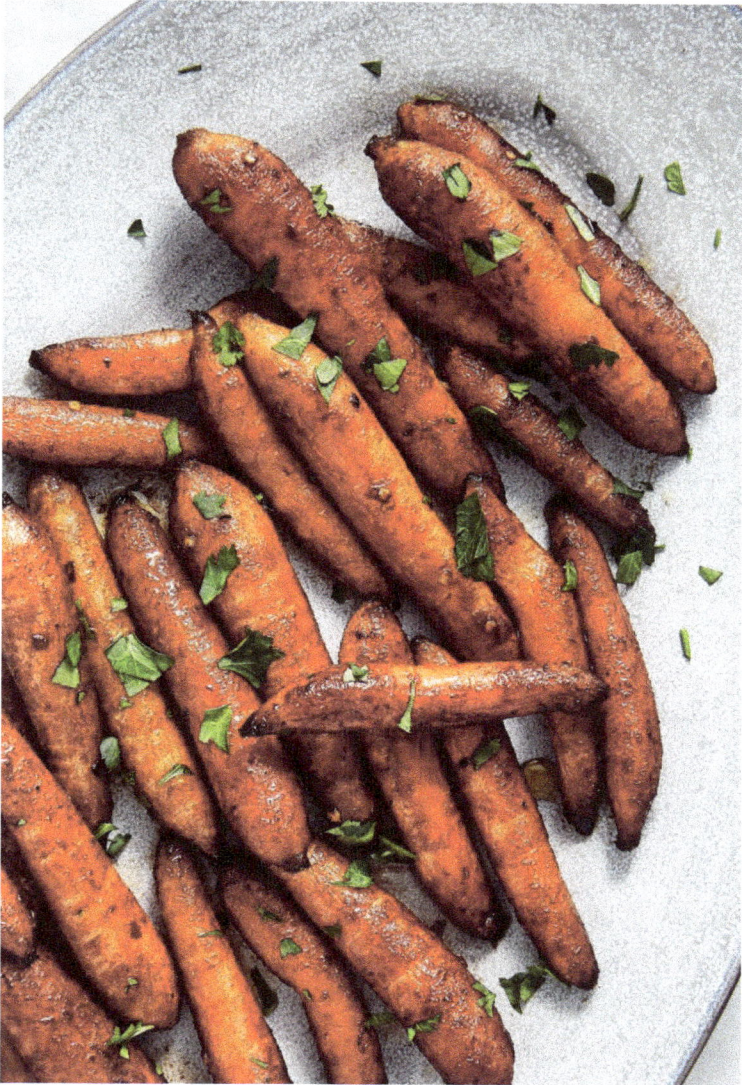

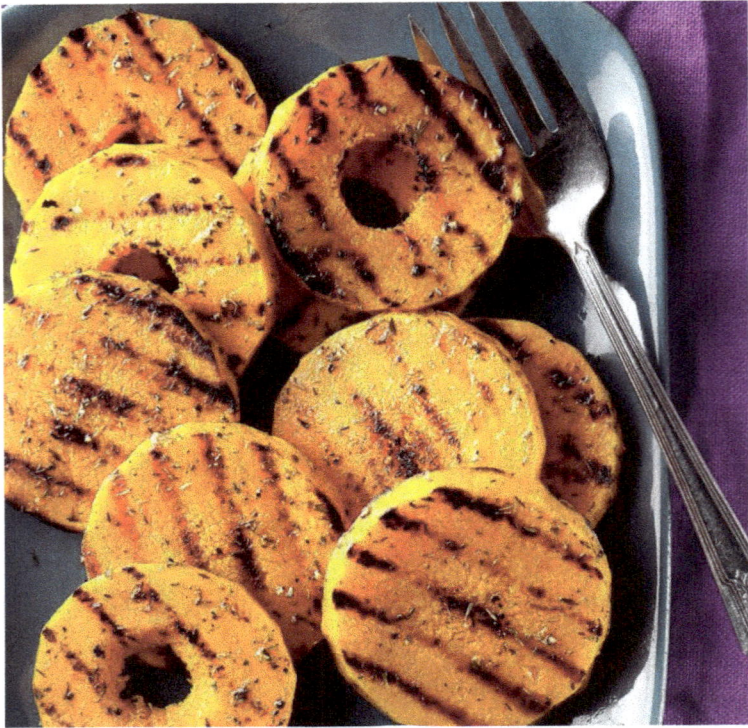

Ingredients

- 1 winter squash, peeled and sliced lengthwise

- ½ cup baby carrots

- 1 bunch of turnip greens

- 2 large red onions, cut into ½ inch rings but don't separate into individual rings

Dressing Ingredients

- 6 tbsp. extra virgin olive oil

- Sea salt, to taste

- 3 tbsp. Balsamic vinegar

- 1 tsp. Dijon mustard

Directions:

Marinate the vegetable with the dressing or marinade ingredients for 15 to 30 min. Grill for 4 minutes over medium heat or until the vegetable becomes tender

Grilled Beetroots and Artichoke Hearts in Viniagrette

Ingredients

- 1 cup canned artichoke hearts
- 2 beetroots, peeled and sliced lengthwise

Dressing Ingredients

- 6 tbsp. olive oil
- Sea salt, to taste
- 3 tbsp. white wine vinegar
- 1 tsp. English mustard

Directions:

Marinate the vegetable with the dressing or marinade ingredients for 15 to 30 min. Grill for 4 minutes over medium heat or until the vegetable becomes tender.

Grilled Beetroots Artichoke Hearts and Asparagus

Ingredients

- ½ cup canned artichoke hearts

- 2 beetroots, peeled and sliced lengthwise

- 10 pcs. Asparagus

Dressing Ingredients

- 6 tbsp. extra virgin olive oil

- Sea salt, to taste

- 3 tbsp. apple cider vinegar

- 1 tbsp. honey

- 1 tsp. Egg-free mayonnaise

Directions:

Marinate the vegetable with the dressing or marinade ingredients for 15 to 30 min. Grill for 4 minutes over medium heat or until the vegetable becomes tender.

Grilled Summer Squash with Balsamic Glaze

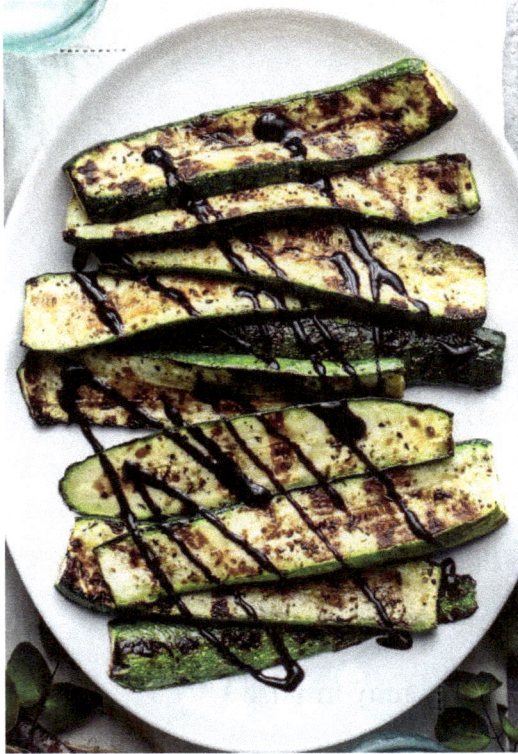

Ingredients

- 1 summer squash, peeled and sliced lengthwise

Dressing Ingredients

- 6 tbsp. extra virgin olive oil

- Sea salt, to taste

- 3 tbsp. Balsamic vinegar

- 1 tsp. Dijon mustard

Directions:

Marinate the vegetable with the dressing or marinade ingredients for 15 to 30 min. Grill for 4 minutes over medium heat or until the vegetable becomes tender.

www.ingramcontent.com/pod-product-compliance
Lightning Source LLC
Chambersburg PA
CBHW071108030426
42336CB00013BA/1997